Praise for the First Edition of

"This is a very important book that bedside of many, many couples."

—Pat Love Ph.D.
Co-author of *Hot Monogamy*

"This forthright and clearly written guide, written by a prostate cancer survivor and his partner, will help men and their partners understand what affects sexual function and how to fix what is in need of repair."

—Stephen B. Strum, M.D.,
Prostate Oncologist and
Director, Prostate Cancer Research Institute

"This book ventures down a road where only the brave dare tread. It will help transform victims into loving individuals with a renewed zest for living."

—Jess Rifkind
Prostate cancer survivor

"This book is an invaluable resource for prostate cancer survivors and their partners dealing with impotence."

—Richard J. Howe
Survivor and activist

"This is a straightforward and practical book offering cancer survivors and their partners a way to begin again after cancer."

—Jane Reese-Coulbourne
Former Executive Vice Pesident,
National Breast Cancer Coalition

"My wife and I are grateful for the work Ralph and Barbara Alterowitz have done and for the encouragement it provides couples like us. I recommend it, however, to all couples who want or need to reinvigorate their relationship with loving sexual and emotional intimacy."

—Herbie Mann
Prostate cancer survivor

"Excellent advice! Unquestionably helps prostate cancer patients and survivors."

—Charles Troshinsky, M.D.
Psychiatrist and prostate cancer survivor

"This book should be most helpful to many couples involved with this dreadful disease. I particularly like the upbeat tone."

—Walter Schiff
Prostate cancer survivor

"Practical advice that applies to all relationships, not just to prostate patients. Presented candidly, but in a way that doesn't make me feel that I have to read it under the covers with a flashlight."

—Bill Cusack
Prostate cancer activist

"Commitment, caring, and the mutual desire to keep the fire of love burning—these are at the heart of this book. This book is a must-read not only for cancer patients affected by disease or treatment, but for everyone."

—Israel Barken, M.D.
Urological Oncologist and
President, Prostate Cancer Research and Education Foundation

"This is a practical guide to help couples reestablish and enhance their sexual relationship when medical or psychological issues have gotten in the way of sexual functioning."

—Chris Kraft, Ph.D.
Instructor and Psychologist,
Johns Hopkins Center for Sexual Health and Medicine

Intimacy with Impotence

The Couple's Guide to Better Sex after Prostate Disease

Ralph and Barbara Alterowitz

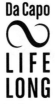

Da Capo

LIFE
LONG

A Member of the Perseus Books Group

Copyright © 2004 by Ralph and Barbara Alterowitz

Originally published in 1999 as *The Lovin' Ain't Over.*

All rights reserved. No part of this publication may be reproduced, stored in a retrieval system, or transmitted, in any form or by any means, electronic, mechanical, photocopying, recording, or otherwise, without the prior written permission of the publisher.

Designed by Inkwell Publishing Services. Set in 11-point Stone Serif by Inkwell Publishing Services.

Library of Congress Cataloging-in-Publication Data

Alterowitz, Ralph.
   Intimacy with impotence : the couple's guide to better sex after prostate disease / Ralph and Barbara Alterowitz.—1st Da Capo Press ed.
      p. cm.
   Includes bibliographical references and index.
   ISBN 978-0-7382-0789-6 (pbk. : alk. paper)
   1. Impotence.   2. Sex.   3. Sex instruction.   4. Prostate-Cancer-Complications.   5. Prostate-Cancer-Patients-Sex behavior.   I. Alterowitz, Barbara.   II. Title.
   RC889.A459 2004
   616.6′922—dc22
                                                                2004003398

First Da Capo Lifelong Books edition 2004
Published by Da Capo Lifelong Books
A Member of the Perseus Books Group
http://www.dacapopress.com

Da Capo Lifelong books are available at special discounts for bulk purchases in the U.S by corporations, institutions, and other organizations. For more information, please contact the Special Markets Department at the Perseus Books Group, 11 Cambridge Center, Cambridge, MA 02142, or call (800) 255-1514 or (617) 252-5298, or e-mail *special.markets@perseusbooks.com.*

Contents

Foreword

Discussing the topics of erection, intimacy, and love requires overcoming personal barriers and social taboos that almost assure that communication is dampened or denied. Just recall the last time you discussed these issues publicly or in a serious manner. The lack of thoughtful books directed to those confronting intimacy and sexual difficulties underscores the need for these issues to be addressed by patients who have experienced such problems and who have sought information and solutions.

There are many approaches, and results can vary. Everyone with the same recipe cannot bake the same cake. However, even though the approaches and outcomes may vary, each couple faces many common problems and decisions. Some guideposts help as we traverse through life's complex and sensitive paths. Certainly medical advice is central, but so are the experiences and perspectives of the patients and their partners.

Ralph and Barbara Alterowitz have collected some of these important guideposts and, with common sense and good judgment, have illuminated them for the layperson. They have presented the issues in a clear and informative manner. Where else are these issues addressed, survivor to survivor, in such a delicate and compassionate manner? The Alterowitz's have made a pioneering effort to illuminate this topic in a sensitive manner, and they will be thanked by the many who will say, "Thank goodness for *Intimacy with Impotence.*"

—DONALD S. COFFEY, Ph.D.
Professor and Director of Urological Research
The Johns Hopkins Medical Institution

Preface

This book is not "The Ralph and Barbara story," although the idea for it originally sprang from our own experiences. Rather, it is meant as a practical guide to help cancer survivors and their partners who are dealing with erectile dysfunction. Like you, we are living the experience. So we are talking to you as patient to patient, partner to partner. This is a book from us to other couples who have survived prostate cancer or other male pelvic diseases and whose normal sexual function has been disrupted. We hope it will help you restore intimacy, and rebuild and improve your love life and sexuality.

When a couple faces erectile dysfunction, they have three choices: One is to end their sex life. The second is to try the aids and medications available to treat erectile dysfunction, keep their fingers crossed, and hope for the best (though in most cases they will find that it's not really the same, even with the medications). The third choice is to transform their love life into a deeply satisfying emotional and sexual relationship by consciously changing the way they make love and not relying entirely on aids and medications.

It is for the third group, and to some extent the second group, that this book is written. We discuss aids and medications extensively, but we hope that we can open many couples' minds to the fact that they can have fabulous erection-free sex. Lovemaking will be different from how it used to be, but it can be wonderful, and it can free you from the obsession with the erection.

Ten years ago, our life plan did not include the idea that we would discuss sexuality and intimacy in public. But life had a surprise in store for us: In 1995, Ralph was diagnosed with prostate cancer. His treatment was successful, and we stayed involved in the prostate cancer community. Many support group meetings later, it became clear that impotence was a major quality-of-life issue for many survivors. We began to read and research the issue, partially for the support group discussions and partially because we ourselves were working through the issues posed by erectile dysfunction.

There was almost no literature on the subject for the lay person, but Ralph, having an extensive biology and medical background, was able to translate the medical jargon. Soon we found ourselves talking to support groups about sexual intimacy and eventually wrote the book, *The Lovin' Ain't Over*. Though it was marketed almost exclusively by word of mouth, the book just kept selling—and readers told us they found it very valuable. Four years later, there were so many new developments in the field that we were approached to update the book.

In addition to the new medications now available or under development, we have added a discussion of off label uses of medications (doctors' use of FDA-approved medication for purposes other than those the drug was approved for). Other new sections were added on talking with your partner and talking with your doctor. The original sections were also updated to reflect additional research and our learnings from many discussions with other couples and individuals.

For us, dealing with erectile dysfunction opened the door to gain a deeper understanding of each other and to revitalize our relationship. Many other couples have gone through a similar process and found that their relationship is stronger than ever—emotionally and physically. For many people, it is not easy to take the first step. As Chaim Potok said in his book, *In the Beginning*, "Be patient. You are learning a new way of understanding. ... All beginnings are hard."

The goal makes it worthwhile: to have a strong, loving, exciting relationship, and to have great sensual sex as a way to keep you connected as a couple.

Good luck and good health.

—RALPH AND BARBARA ALTEROWITZ

Acknowledgments

This book could not have been written without our interaction with thousands of survivors and partners. This is their book. They are the motivating force behind the book. In our *The Lovin' Ain't Over* sessions and in counseling, they asked us to write this book for all couples who have erectile dysfunction and intimacy problems. They also provided much of the information. We've painted their stories of pain, disappointment, and success in reviving intimacy in this book.

Physicians, researchers, psychologists, and pharmaceutical companies and manufacturers contributed material and made suggestions to help couples after seeing the value of the first book. All of them reviewed the book or specific sections to make sure the information was objective, accurate, current, and validated.

Much is owed to Dr. Christopher Kraft of The Johns Hopkins Medical Institution Sexual and Marital Therapy. With him we explored the nature of intimacy and sexual difficulties in relationships and came up with original ways to help people work through their problems.

Certainly the section on medical therapies and medications would have been deficient without the counseling and information provided by Dr. Arthur Burnett, Professor of Urology and Director, Male Sexual Health Clinic, Johns Hopkins Medical Institution. It would be difficult to find as knowledgeable a clinician, with his experience as a surgeon, erectile dysfunction specialist, and researcher into erectile therapies.

Pharmaceutical companies and device manufacturers provided current information on their products and research and then reviewed the accuracy of the information we prepared. The companies are included in the List of Contributors.

To take all this and make it readable is a tough job. We are fortunate because we have Jon Zonderman, who can make music out of the notes he gets. He usually collaborates with Ralph on his business books, but agreed to work with us again on this topic. As with other books, he helped with structuring this book and, as always, added considerable clarity to our writing. He also provided valuable insights on the topic of off label medication use based on his research for other health-related books.

Without Dr. Carol Partington, this book would not have become a reality. She did the painstaking research on the medications, obtained input from the manufacturers, and participated in the writing. Her calm and reassuring presence was a stable core in the often maddening process of researching and writing a book, and her wealth of knowledge and understanding of the medical issues resolved many questions. Without her, we could not have made the deadline for publication.

On the patient and partner side, we owe much to so many people. Special thanks go to Philip and Margaret Brach, to April and Larry Becker, and to Steve and Betsy Corman for their thoughts and contributions. We are also grateful for the many support group coordinators who give so freely of their time to help cancer patients, and for the support and advice of James Lewis, Ph.D.

To bring this book out we were fortunate to find in Gail Ross, our agent, a believer who felt that prostate cancer couples needed this updated edition. When Marnie Cochran became our editor, little did we know the gem she would be. Little is usually written about copy editors, but we would be remiss in not recognizing Fred Dahl, whose suggestions improved both the text and graphics.

The experience of Ralph's cancer and recovery has been a spiritual journey as much as it was a medical and psychological one. We do not take our life or our love for granted. They are gifts we treasure and are thankful for.

—Barbara and Ralph Alterowitz

List of Contributors

Principal Contributors

Dr. Arthur L. Burnett, M.D., FACS
Professor of Urology and Director, Male Sexual Health Clinic
The Johns Hopkins Medical Institution—for contributions to the
  Therapies and Medications

Chris Kraft, Ph.D.
Center for Marital and Sexual Health,
Sexual Behaviors Consultation Unit
The Johns Hopkins Medical Institution—for contributions to
  improving the quality of marital relationships

Other Contributors

Dr. John P. Mulhall, M.D.
Director, Sexual Medicine Programs, Department of Urology
Weill Medical College of Cornell University
New York Presbyterian Hospital and Memorial Sloan Kettering
  Center

Dr. J. Douglas Trapp, M.D.
President, Impotence Consultant Service, Inc.

Stanley E. Althof, Ph.D.
Department of Urology Psychology, Case Western Reserve
  University School of Medicine and Center for Marital and
  Sexual Health

Pharmaceutical Companies and Device Manufacturers

American Medical Systems—Web site: *www.visitams.com*
American MedTech—Web site: *www.rejoyn.com*

Augusta Medical Systems—Web site: *www.augustams.com*
Bayer—Web site: www.bayer.com
Encore Medical Products—Web site: *www.impoaid.com*
Lilly—Web site: *www.cialis.com*
MacroChem—Web site: *www.macrochem.com*
Mentor Corp.—Web site: *www.mentorcorp.com*
Mission Pharmacal—Web site: *www.missionpharmacal.com*
NexMed—Web site: *www.nexmed.com*
Palatin Technologies, Inc.—Web site: *www.palatin.com*
Pfizer—Web site: *www.viagra.com*
Pfizer (formerly Pharmacia-Upjohn)—Web site: *www.caverject.com*
Pos-T-Vac—Web site: *www.postvac.com*
Schwarz Pharma—Web site: *www.schwarzusa.com*
Senetek—Web site: *www.senetekplc.com*
TAP Pharmaceutical Products, Inc.—Web site: *www.tap.com*
TIMM Medical Technologies (a subsidiary of Endocare, Inc.)—
    Web site: *www.timmmedical.com*
VIVUS, Inc.—Web site: *www.vivus.com*
Zonagen—Web site: *www.zonagen.com*

Additional Information and Updates

If you enjoyed this book and found it helpful, more information
is availble at:

www.renewintimacy.org or *www.thelovinaintover.org*

If you have comments or questions for Ralph and Barbara
Alterowitz, please email them to: *ralph@renewintimacy.org* or
barbara@renewintimacy.org.

If you would like to be notified about future updates to this
book, please send your name, address, phone number, and email
address to:

IWI
P.O. Box 341388
Bethesda, MD 20827-1388

Introduction

With *Intimacy with Impotence* (the updated version of *The Lovin' Ain't Over*), Ralph and Barbara Alterowitz have given me another privileged opportunity to write the Introduction. The edition is most timely since it continues to bring attention to two important matters: sexual health and prostate cancer. For the former, there is now widespread recognition that sexual function is not a taboo subject with mythical associations but rather a vitally important aspect of normal life. For the latter, prostate cancer remains the most commonly diagnosed malignancy among men in the United States, having particular impact with regard to consequences of its management: that sexual function may be lost or reduced by the appropriate treatment. This issue is a serious consideration for many men, discouraging them from undergoing screening for the diagnosis of prostate cancer and its subsequent treatment. For many men, the predicament of living longer but maybe not better may lead them to ignore the possibility of having the disease. For some men, retaining sexual function becomes more important than undergoing treatment for a life-threatening disease, a process that threatens this function. This issue is clearly agonizing and possibly handled best with the type of tongue-in-cheek humor expressed by one of my patients: "I have come to the determination that the ultimate form of sexual dysfunction is death, and so I should proceed with your recommendations for treatment." Indeed, while successful eradication of malignancy is most certainly the primary goal of treatment for prostate cancer, preserving sexual function is a substantial and worthy secondary objective.

As in the first edition, this book identifies the importance of preserving sexual health as a major component of overall health.

It further assigns a critical role to sexual function recovery after prostate cancer treatment for maintaining an overall sense of well-being among cancer survivors. This perspective impresses on all concerned with treating prostate cancer—medical professionals and lay public individuals alike—the charge to improve on current goals of therapy beyond just life preservation. Extended goals include the purpose of restoring a couple's well-being and the quality of life imparted by a healthy and fulfilling sexual life. The main emphasis of *Intimacy with Impotence* centers on the positive interaction of a couple's relationship. This interaction applies to dealing with the difficulties and emotions of the prostate cancer diagnosis and treatment. It also applies to regaining and strengthening the experience of lovemaking in the context of the relationship. I consider this emphasis a particularly meritorious aspect of the book and a concept that we medical professionals should fully learn from our patients: that restoring the function of the sexual organ should be combined with the roles of communication, trust, and intimacy for a maximally satisfying sexual experience.

This current edition remains highly informative and educational. Since the field of sexual medicine has rapidly evolved in recent years, the book offers an accurate review of current treatment options for preserving, restoring, and promoting sexual health. Also included is information regarding new directions in the field that offer further promise for men who must agonize over the prospect of lost sexual ability with prostate cancer treatment.

I congratulate again Ralph and Barbara Alterowitz for their accomplishment. It is clear that they understand fully the impact of prostate cancer treatment and the purpose of helping others to get through this experience positively.

—Arthur L. Burnett, M.D., FACS
Professor of Urology
Director, Male Sexual Health Clinic
The Johns Hopkins Medical Institution

Impotence: An Opportunity to Revive Intimacy

Key Points

✔ *Sexuality is an essential aspect of intimacy, and intimacy is the foundation of a loving relationship.*

✔ *Sex is more than intercourse.*

✔ *The only thing a couple loses when impotence strikes is the ability for penetration. Both partners can still have desire, arousal, sexual touching, orgasm, and sexual pleasure and satisfaction.*

✔ *A broad range of activities can compensate for varying degrees of impotence.*

✔ *Both partners must work together to achieve a mutually satisfying experience.*

✔ *A good relationship is the foundation for good loving. There are many ways to move from a RUT marriage (Routine, Unappreciated, and Tired) to a CREST marriage (characterized by Creativity, Respect, Excitement, Sensitivity, and Togetherness).*

✔ *Erectile dysfunction means change and an opportunity to revitalize a couple's relationship and lovemaking.*

Think back to when you or your partner were first diagnosed. What did you focus on when you were first told that you (or your partner) had cancer? If you are like us and many others, your first thought was about survival. Then, after treatment started or when the first round of therapy was over and imminent death was no longer the immediate issue, your thoughts turned to other questions: "How normal can our lives be, even if the cancer is under control? And what about sex?"

Given that prostate, bladder, and colorectal cancers generally affect people over fifty, it is safe to say that most of us grew up at a time when sex, loving, and parts of our anatomy were not as openly discussed as they are today. When we were kids we didn't talk about loving. Boys' "locker room" conversations were about sex. Women, when they were girls, talked about love. Girls who "did it" were not "nice." Everyone had heard the expression—"Nice girls don't."

Despite more open discussion of sex today, the world hasn't come very far in terms of connecting sex with love.

Is it any wonder that after therapy for prostate, bladder, or colorectal cancer, which makes men impotent to one degree or another, many or most couples do not talk about sex? They continue to treat the subject as taboo. By avoiding the subject, they build one of the biggest barriers to overcoming the problem.

Reality Hits

Even before surgical or radiation therapy for cancer of the prostate, bladder, or colon, most men lose some of their sexual capability after fifty. Although they would like to believe that they were performing almost as well sexually before cancer therapy as they did when they were twenty, unfortunately this is not the case.

Men have a Lake Woebegonesque mental image of their sexual capability; just like the people who inhabit Garrison Keillor's mythical town, they are all "above average." When filling out the sex questionnaire at the doctor's office, we may have flashed back to our younger days and written that our erections were steel-hard and that we had sex at least three times a week. But the reality is that most of us were already well into the gray zone, somewhere between our twenties' level of potency and our fifties' level of impotence (before we were treated for cancer). For some, a lifestyle of stress, smoking, and eating fatty foods had already led to the blockage of arteries, which does the same to the penis as to the heart. Even for those with a relatively healthy lifestyle, age-related deterioration of sexual capacity was setting in.

Whatever your level of erectile function, cancer therapy can make things worse in two ways. First is the psychological component. After you get the blow of the cancer diagnosis, you find out that the treatment will affect your potency. Second is the physical and physiological consequences of the treatments, which highlight any underlying erectile dysfunction.

Common misconceptions can actually worsen erectile dysfunction. In his 1998 *Geriatrics* article, "Erectile dysfunction: A practical approach for primary care," Dr. Arthur Burnett, Director of the Male Sexual Health Clinic at Johns Hopkins Medical Institution, wrote: "Erectile dysfunction carries the implication of sexual failure and is associated with anxiety, depression, marital discord, and even violence."

The FDA approval of and subsequent marketing of Viagra® in 1998 seems to have been a major event that spurred men to get help. An early Pfizer study found that, after Viagra® became available, twice as many men with erectile dysfunction went for counseling.

Cancer therapy reduces sexual capability as measured by the ability to get an erection, the rigidity of erections, and how long the erections last. However, there are many therapies and medications available to help men improve their ability. But couples need to take the initiative to overcome the problem. Some men expect that, after cancer treatment, their erections will be as good or even better than they were before. In truth, even with treatment for erectile dysfunction, capability is usually less, and, in the best case, erections are only almost as good as before treatment.

Treatment for prostate, bladder, or colorectal cancer is a "focusing event." You can use it to redefine and refine the sexual aspects of your relationship and put the issue of impotence in a context of intimacy that is more complex and subtle than dealing with the cancer itself.

So we'll ask the question: What do men want? If your answer is a happy satisfying love life for both partners, then read on. You are now a member of the brotherhood and sisterhood of surviving couples who recognize that intimacy and sexuality are essential to their relationship. When it comes to intimacy, cancer treatment that causes some degree of impotence is a wake-up call *to motivate you to change your habits in your love life to revive your intimacy.* It's a golden opportunity for the partners to work together toward *a much better love life for both of you.*

This book describes the steps a couple can take to resume a healthy and happy sex life. The key is to create a different pattern of behavior for loving. The point is that, given the problems a couple has following any treatment that results in potency difficulties for the man, they can look on developing a different pattern for loving as another means of dealing with the situation—in other words, something akin to another therapy. Many therapies and medications deal with the erectile dysfunction part of the problem. But it is essential to know that the man's ability to have an erection does not always mean that the couple, or even the man, will have a satisfactory sex life. Sex and the erection must mesh into the partners' relationship with each other.

Even before cancer treatment, few men in midlife and older could be instantaneous sex partners. They as well as their partners needed warmup, arousal time. Getting sexually excited takes much longer considering the damage done to nerves and blood vessels by surgery, radiation, cryoablation, hormone treatment, or any combination of these therapies. If a couple renews its sexual foundation, loving can be as good as or better than it was previously.

Good sex requires partners to let themselves go and get completely immersed in the loving. Both men and women need to feel comfortable with each other to engage in sex. It takes trust and a willingness to consider and try new things.

Relearning to make love makes your relationship new and exciting. You discover new things; you behave differently; you see sides of your partner that delight and surprise you. It's almost like having an affair with your current partner—and you don't have to feel one bit of guilt!

We are more capable than previous generations of making these changes. According to a 1973 survey (when most of us midlifers were between twenty-five and forty-five), we had already made major breaks from the sexual patterns of our parents.

From Relationship RUT to CREST

After a number of years many marriages are stuck in the *RUT*: The relationship becomes *R*outine, *U*nappreciated, and *T*ired. Partners often do not appreciate each other or the relationship, and there is an underlying tiredness in the marriage. Areas in a marriage cannot be separated from each other. Any difficulties in one part of the relationship affect all other areas.

The pressures of everyday life continually force the priorities to be reordered. And for many, sex drops to a lower priority. You may not get "turned on" by your partner as much anymore, and living with her (or him) may have become routine. The situation is what psychologists call *habituation*. Patricia Love, Ed.D., author of *Hot Monogamy*, has a colorful way of putting it: "If you live by the railroad tracks and a train goes by, you don't even wake up." As one long married wife put it: "A lot of things fall by the wayside when you're married awhile."

But how do you get to a *CREST* relationship, where the relationship is characterized by *C*reativity, *R*espect, *E*xcitement, *S*ensitivity, and *T*ogetherness? Judith S. Wallerstein, in her book *The Good Marriage: How and Why Love Lasts*, says, "a good sex life, however the couple defines that, is at the heart of a good marriage." She says that sexual love is one of the nine fundamental characteristics of a good marriage. "This is the domain where intimacy is renewed, and the excitement that first drew the couple together is kept alive. ... There is no better antidote to the pressures of living than a loving sex life." Some recent studies even say that sex increases longevity.

Rather than cancer treatment closing the door to physical intimacy, a constructive approach to impotence problems can expose a couple to new possibilities and experiences that will enrich their relationship. It means that the partners must open themselves to a new perspective of what loving is all about, broaden their communications, and see ways for introducing flexibility in their respective styles of loving. Introducing newness into your lovemaking can energize you and increase your enthusiasm. In this book, we will look at some of the many factors that bear on this.

This book is about love in a relationship. That means we must talk about communication, shared experiences, joint involvement, and, of course, intimacy.

Gail Sheehy defines the capacity for intimacy as "the art of giving to another while still maintaining a lively sense of self." In other words, for each of us, our capacity for intimacy is being able to be me, you, and us. Each partner has to express his or her own personality, needs, and desires during lovemaking, while simultaneously being thoughtful and sensitive to the needs of his or her partner.

The basic premise for this discussion is that *you can have a loving and satisfying sexual relationship without having an erection.* We'll give you tips on therapies, devices, and medication for getting an erection, but we urge you not to focus on the erection. You'll both have much more fun and satisfaction if you avoid doing that.

Breaking the Erectile Dysfunction Mindset

Erectile dysfunction means CHANGE *in lifestyle and lovemaking.* Regardless of the reasons that lessen a man's capability to have an erection, his feelings about himself and his relationship with his partner will change.

Knowing that it will not be the same anymore, men go through emotions of anger, rejection, and depression. However, many studies have shown that having a positive outlook helps in getting through any difficult medical condition. In a study of more than twenty-two thousand adults in Finland, investigators found that men with high levels of satisfaction in their lives lived longer.

The *Positive Aging* newsletter notes, "the meaning we assign to biological events may have significant implications for the course they take. To illustrate, some victims of a heart attack draw meaning from the event ... to have a deeper appreciation of life." One study found that "men who were able to find some positive meaning in their heart attacks were less likely to have a subsequent one than those who did not ... ." The same is true when it comes to erectile dysfunction. Focusing on the entire loving package rather than on the erection will relieve a man's anxiety over whether he will get an erection and enable him to enjoy other parts of loving.

Cancer survivors continually have reminders that cancer is part of their lives in news reports, in periodic lab tests, and for some in the products they use daily, such as incontinence pads. A constant reminder of cancer for almost every survivor of prostate, bladder, or colorectal cancer is the bedroom. For them, erections are usually hard to get naturally, if they are gotten at all.

We cannot prevent cancer from becoming a life changing event. At one support group meeting, one man asked, "Is there life after prostate cancer?" Looking for what comes next begins with the man's option to accept the life event as just another life event; then he can open himself to possibilities that can make life more meaningful.

One man went back to tennis and golf in spite of his extreme incontinence. For him, doing what he wanted was living. Sure, it meant some things had to change. But it was either that or forget part of the life he wanted to have. It may sound simple, but it isn't. Quality living has always been an art form. Some people master it better than others.

So much of every man's life is bound up with his partner and his family that one area of concentration should be making that relationship as strong as possible. Physical intimacy is a key and major part of it. We say "physical intimacy" because some couples will see it as including loving and others not. For some, loving and sex are the same and others will break it down further. Whatever your definition, successful loving makes you happy with the physical contact you have. It may or may not include penetration, you may or may not have orgasms all the time, but you can feel good all the time. In each relationship, the partners must decide mutually what they want.

Back to the Subject of Sex:
Happiness Is an Erection—or Is It?

Happiness is an erection! That's what many men with erection problems would like to believe at first. And there are lots of therapies to help them get erections. Since many therapies work well, why do many men stop taking them? Somewhere between fifty and seventy-five percent of men who have been treated for erectile dysfunction stop using the therapies prescribed. What is going on here?

Giving up is understandable when a given treatment or several treatments do not work. The man and his partner may decide not to go further to find one that achieves the desired results. Yet, given the presumed importance of erections, one would expect that almost all men would continue searching for an effective treatment.

The bigger mystery is why men who have found a successful treatment that enables them to have an erection discontinue using the treatment. Doctors report that these men do not return for treatment refills. Obviously there is more to a satisfying sex life than regaining the erection.

Dr. Stanley E. Althof helps men with intimacy problems. He captured the essence of his findings in the title of an article "When an erection alone is not enough: Biopsychosocial obstacles to love-making." In the article he states: "Giving men firm erections is relatively straightforward these days: getting them to make use of it regularly in lovemaking is more complicated." He talks about what else might be going on that accounts for the high dropout rate. In simple cases, he says, a pill will usually increase a man's capability for sex. But many situations are not so straightforward and factors that can interfere with the successful resumption of lovemaking include "poorly managed or unresolved anger, power and control issues, and contempt and disappointment." Dr. Althof says that quite often these difficulties may be complicated by such factors as:

1. the length of time the couple had not had sex before resuming;
2. the man's approach to resuming a sexual life with his partner;
3. the partner's physical and emotional readiness to resume love-making;
4. the man's expectations of how the medications (e.g., Viagra®) will change his life;
5. the meaning for each partner of using a medication or device;
6. whether there are any unconventional sexual arousal patterns in the man; and

7. the quality of the couple's nonsexual relationship

Based on these questions, we defined a six-step plan that can help a couple improve their physical intimacy (in all forms of physical interaction) and have satisfying, even outstanding sex. This is shown in Figure 1-1. By improving their sexuality, a couple can move closer to a CREST relationship.

Figure 1-1

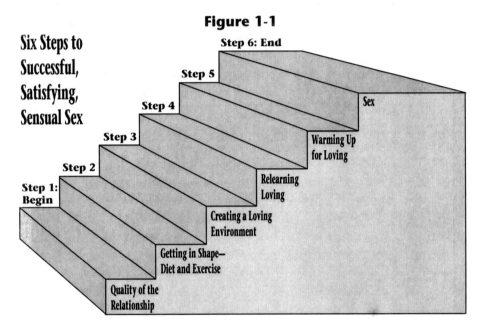

Six Steps to Successful, Satisfying, Sensual Sex

Step 1: Begin — Quality of the Relationship
Step 2 — Getting in Shape—Diet and Exercise
Step 3 — Creating a Loving Environment
Step 4 — Relearning Loving
Step 5 — Warming Up for Loving
Step 6: End — Sex

Great, satisfying, successful sex does not just happen, at least for middle-aged and older people. Successful satisfying sex is based on the emotional, physiological, and the physical parts coming together. Great sex, or even average sex, requires a foundation.

Our sex cannot be the impromptu, spur-of-the-moment sex that young people can have. Their physical intimacy may not be the result of deep emotional bonding. Many people contend that sex has a richer aspect when it arises from long-term relationships in which partners have developed the many points of connection over time. These bonds provide the substance that draw the partners ever closer and foster the desire they feel for each other.

Mindset

As in any area that is worth pursuing and doing, including loving, it takes learning, time, patience, and practice to do it well. We may want the practice but we need the other parts of the loving package to have great sex. As Sophia Loren said, sexiness begins in the head and then it goes somewhere else.

After cancer treatment, men have to think differently about sex. Thinking of it as making love might be a start. This is a different way of thinking about sex than men have been accustomed to. When we were younger, the transmission of thought and the processing of various stimuli (a pretty woman, a certain smell, a pair of beautiful legs) all led almost instantaneously to an erection.

Now, getting an erection requires men to do some things. And sometimes the erection does not come even with a medication that may have worked the time before. But if in thinking differently about sex, the man is prepared to enjoy other parts of loving as well, then having the erection won't count for as much. After all, if the physical connection with the partner and the feelings associated with it are really the objective, then the erection is just one means for achieving it. That and an orgasm can still be had.

Couples who have successfully built a new sex life with impotence realize that an erection is not required for good sex. They have learned to give sexual pleasure to each other in many ways, with and without medication. The process of relearning loving has revitalized their relationship, and they have found that freeing themselves from the obsession with the erection has liberated them to try new things together, be creative, and learn more about their own and their partner's sexuality. In so doing, they find they have deepened their emotional intimacy.

Facts about Impotence

Key Points

✔ *Many physical factors cause impotence, but impotence need not prevent a couple from having a good love life.*

✔ *Men can't control accidents, disease, or injuries, but they can keep alcohol, drugs, and smoking from ruining their sex life.*

✔ *There is no prescribed "normal frequency" for lovemaking; each couple defines "normal" for themselves.*

✔ *Erectile dysfunction is not a yes-or-no condition; there are many levels of potency.*

✔ *Men's delay in arousal as they get older brings them more in tune with women.*

✔ *It's okay, normal, and healthy to make love as one gets older. Loving and sex are measures of the health of a relationship and the health of each partner.*

✔ *Most prostate cancer patients (and many survivors of other cancers in the pelvic area) experience some degree of erectile dysfunction.*

✔ *After prostate cancer surgery, it's hard to tell immediately what the new "natural" level of potency will be. Sometimes it takes more than two years to recover potency.*

✔ *Men and women can have orgasms without erections.*

✔ *Erection medications do not work on everyone and may not work equally well each time a person takes them.*

We use the two terms *impotence* and *erectile dysfunction (ED)* interchangeably. Impotence is a man's inability to obtain and maintain an erection sufficient for intercourse. Unfortunately, people tend to think of impotence as if it indicates a total and irrevocable condition. In reality, there are different levels of erectile dysfunction, or impotence, and many of them can be addressed.

Causes of Erectile Dysfunction

Erectile function is affected by some things men have control over and by other things men have no control over. In addition to cancer therapy, erectile dysfunction can be caused by accidents, injury, or disease. In some instances, even medications can cause or worsen erectile dysfunction.

About a dozen chronic diseases cause varying degrees of impotence. Diabetes is responsible for about forty percent of all cases of impotence; vascular and heart disease for about thirty percent; radical surgery for about thirteen percent; spinal injury for about eight percent; and endocrine disorders for about six percent.

Some of these conditions are made worse by lifestyle, and all are complicated by the effects of aging. The three major lifestyle causes of erectile dysfunction are:

- *Alcohol:* People talk of going out to eat and drink and then making love. While a little alcohol (a glass of wine or a beer) can decrease anxiety and inhibition and generally relax a person, more than this acts as a sedative. Several drinks are likely to make a person sleepy and less able to actively participate in sex. In many men, alcohol reduces the ability to have an erection and an orgasm.

- *Street and prescription drugs:* A range of prescription drugs available today lessen the ability and the energy to make love. Some drugs, both prescription and street drugs, increase desire and a sense of sensuality, but *decrease* erectile function.

Prescription drugs include those prescribed to cope with and control cardiovascular problems such as hypertension and angina, anxiety, depression, psychosis, and other conditions. For example, finasteride, sold under the names of Proscar and

Propecia, has been found to prevent or delay prostate cancer in fifteen out of every thousand men taking the drug. It has been used to shrink enlarged prostate glands and fights male baldness. However, a significant side effect is that it can cause impotence.

If you suspect that a prescription drug is causing impotence, ask your doctor if there is an alternative medication that may not have this side effect. If you are taking street drugs, stop immediately. If you are dependent on a drug, seek help if you want to preserve your love life.

• *Smoking:* Research has increasingly shown the direct cause-and-effect relationship between smoking and erectile dysfunction. Nicotine directly interferes with circulation and the pathways of the nervous system, thereby decreasing a man's ability to have good erections. Smoking clogs the small blood vessels in the penis as well as in the heart. Obviously, if the blood vessels are clogged, an erection cannot occur.

Sexuality, Impotence, and Age

With impotence a much more public topic than even four years ago, estimates have begun appearing in health reports that as many as thirty to thirty-five million American men suffer varying degrees of impotence. Men as young as twenty years of age have sought treatment. By the time a man is thirty years old, there is a ten percent chance of having problems attaining or maintaining an erection. About fifty-two percent of men between forty and fifty report that they have had impotence problems. By the time men are in their fifties and sixties, more than half of them have experienced *significant* erectile dysfunction.

What Is a "Normal" Sex Life?

Many people try to measure and quantify everything, including how often they make love. It seems like many of us are searching for the holy grail of sex. But what is "normal"? In November 1998, *The New York Times* said: "Most couples consider good sex vital to a marriage's success, [and] have sex about once a week, for an average of 39 minutes." (While writing this section, we listened to Ravel's "Bolero," considered a very erotic piece of music.

Unfortunately, it has to be played three times to accompany the average American lovemaking session because it's only thirteen minutes long!)

Another survey showed that Americans fall into three groups: One-third have sex twice a week or more, one-third a few times a month, and one-third a few times a year or not at all. In 1973, the average couple (then thirty-five to forty-five years old, today's sixty- to seventy-year-olds) had sex ninety-nine times a year, almost twice weekly.

Even the Viagra® market forecasters could not decide what "normal" is. They prepared revenue forecasts based on a man using the pill from twice a month to as much as twice a week.

The bottom line is: *Normal for you and your partner is whatever gives you both pleasure. Both partners need to agree on how often they should make love to make their life satisfying.*

It's Over—or Is It?

Millions of men have given up on lovemaking because of their erection problems. In the prostate cancer community, one study found that the level of expressed "sexual interest" dropped by half after treatment. Actual sexual activity dropped by almost two-thirds as measured by the "frequency of ... passionate kissing, sexually touching and sexual intercourse," according to *Prostate Cancer and Prostatic Diseases* in a 1998 article.

The physical problems men have are worsened by their "mind trips." They create excuses such as:

• "I'm not interested anymore."
• "I've got other things to do."
• "I'm getting too old."
• "There is nothing I can do about it."
• "What's the point? It won't work anyway."

The fact is that men can continue to have a strong sex drive even if they have erectile dysfunction. It is possible to have good loving for the rest of your life regardless of age, whether you have erectile dysfunction or not. Many men with ED still have some erectile capability. And even without intercourse, you can still have a good love life. It is not necessary to have an erection for either partner to have an orgasm.

It *is* normal to be interested in sex throughout your life. Men and women can remain sexually active throughout their entire lives. No one has to apologize for an interest in sex. Some people believe that sex is only for the young and that as people get older, they lose their desire for sex and their ability to perform. The fact is that we are sexual beings our whole lives. One doctor told us that his eighty-year-old father asked him for a prescription for Viagra®, but asked that he have another doctor in the practice sign the prescription because "your mother doesn't want you to know that we are still having sex." The doctor was delighted because this could mean he would be able to have sex in his eighties.

As men get older, arousal takes longer for a number of reasons. This can be seen as a blessing in disguise because it can make loving much better. In general, women take longer than men to become aroused. Therefore, if a man takes longer to become aroused as well, his partner may be aroused or nearly there by the time he is. This synchronicity of arousal can help both parties to experience the same pleasure during the lovemaking cycle and can remove one of the main complaints younger women have about their love life.

Trollope Works for Me

Before I turn 67 next March I would like to have a lot of sex with a man I like. If you want to talk first, Trollope works for me.

Jane Juska, a sixty-seven-year-old divorced mother of two, placed this personal ad in *The New York Review of Books*, and went on to write a book on what happened after she placed the ad. (In case you're wondering, Trollope was an English novelist in the nineteenth century.)

She and others every day are debunking the myth that older women aren't interested in sex and loving as they get older. That is true for some women, but studies have shown that many women over fifty become more interested in sex because the danger of pregnancy is reduced or gone, and there are fewer family-raising pressures in their lives. In one instance, a woman whose partner introduced her to lubricants at age sixty says she "can't get enough of it [sex]." Again, the only way to find out if your partner is interested is to talk with her.

Since pelvic cancers usually affect older couples, the women in these relationships can end up being deprived of sex when their partners have impotence problems due to cancer treatment. Many men project a lack of interest onto their partners and create other rationales to absolve themselves of the need to make any effort at physical intimacy.

Female partners of pelvic cancer patients complain that their men see impotence as a reason for not having sex. Many women who had good precancer sexual relations are unhappy because their men withdraw due to erectile dysfunction. Some men believe that, if they are incapable of penetration, their partner will see them as less manly and be disappointed by their sexual activity.

Juska writes in her book that by the time she emerged from her chrysalis, she realized she'd never had a chance at pleasure. Similarly, some partners of pelvic cancer patients have not had satisfactory physical intimacy even prior to their partner's treatment for cancer. Often before cancer treatment, the man focused on the erection and penetration—on his own pleasure—and so the loving, nurturing, and caressing the woman finds so important never happened.

Quite often, the self-esteem of a man drops when he has impotence problems. He withdraws, hoping that his partner will retain her former image of him. Sometimes, men use the excuse that they are not having sex anymore because their wife or partner is not interested. Or they believe that, since being treated for prostate cancer, they cannot please their partner.

Certainly, men and their partners do themselves a great disservice and decrease the quality of their lives when they shy away from physical intimacy when in reality both partners want it. Creating artificial blocks and refusing to talk about impotence and intimacy are very damaging behaviors to the relationship. Women can experience close physical intimacy and be highly satisfied even by a totally impotent man. Moreover, men can also achieve sexual satisfaction with any level of erectile dysfunction. But that would mean the man needs to set aside some old concepts that lovemaking can be successful only with a full erection. Maybe it is time to think about making love instead of just having sex.

The Effects of Prostate Cancer Treatment: What's the Truth?

Am I the only one with a problem?

Survivors often assume, "I'm the only one who has a problem. Everyone else came out of therapy okay." The truth is that seventy to ninety percent of prostate cancer survivors have erectile dysfunction *for some time or permanently.*

Leslie Schover, Ph.D., of the Cleveland Clinic Foundation, reported that "the prevalence of sexual problems may be as high as ... 70 percent in prostate cancer survivors." (*Journal of the National Cancer Institute*, Vol. 90, No. 8, April 15, 1998, p. 566). Dr. Schover goes on to note that, "Problems faced by survivors include loss of desire, erectile dysfunction, painful intercourse, and difficulty reaching orgasm."

As many as ninety percent of men who have surgery for prostate cancer will have erectile dysfunction immediately following treatment. Recovery varies widely. One prominent medical center known for prostate surgery estimates that about forty percent of their surgery patients will recover "full function" within six months and about sixty to seventy percent will recover within eighteen months.

A relatively high potency recovery rate may be expected with surgical excellence. The surgeon's skill is an important factor, but not the only one. For instance, recovery for younger men (under sixty) is higher than for older men. However, every procedure results in some loss of erectile capability. The nervous system is like a tree, with large, small, and tiny branches. Even if major nerves are not cut during surgery, some nerves are damaged.

Nerves are also damaged during radiation. When radiation therapy is used, erectile dysfunction appears to be delayed. About twenty to thirty percent of radiation patients have erectile dysfunction right after therapy. Radiation damages the small blood vessels supplying the pelvic region. This leads to fibrosis (scarring that causes toughening) of these small blood vessels. The scarring process builds on itself by interfering with nutrients, blood flow, and oxygenation. In time, the tissue goes from soft to leathery. As a result, within four years after traditional external beam radiation therapy, the percentage of men with erectile dysfunction is the same as among surgery patients. Therefore, although potency is higher in the near term compared with surgery, ultimately the level of impotence resulting from radiation may be comparable to that resulting from surgery. Some new radiation therapies may reduce the likelihood of erectile dysfunction.

Is nerve sparing or nerve grafting surgery a miracle treatment?

One of many prostate cancer myths is this: After a nerve sparing operation the man has the same level of potency as he had before the surgery. We all wish it were true, but it's usually not.

The nerves responsible for erections run alongside the prostate, not through it. They are distributed in the tissue near the prostate gland. Although nerves are not visible to the naked eye, surgeons generally know the surgical landmarks. Therefore if the disease is confined to the gland, it may be possible to spare these areas and preserve some nerves. However, even when the neurovascular bundles are spared, the nerves are traumatized, and many smaller ones are cut.

In 1997, the FDA approved a nerve locating tool, the CaverMap Surgical Aid. UroMed, the manufacturer, said that the patented technology helps surgeons map the microscopic cavernous nerves. The system is currently being used at The Johns Hopkins Medical Institution and other centers of excellence. While the device is still imprecise, more precise technologies may come along now that a breakthrough has been made.

So the doctor does not actually know if the nerve sparing procedure was successful. His or her determination is based only on the observation that "nerves look good at the end of the case."

We know of a support group formed by a number of survivors who were operated on by a prominent surgeon noted for his nerve sparing surgical technique. They shared their experiences and tracked how everyone fared. They found that, although the doctor's self-reported statistics looked good, almost everyone experienced significant erectile dysfunction. Maybe there is a gap between what doctors consider "full function" and what patients perceive as "good."

For the past forty years, the sural nerve in the ankle has been used for radical prostatectomy patients to provide a neural bridge because one or both cavernous nerves were cut. Sural nerve grafting is not a one hundred percent effective technique for retaining potency. Study results show that one-third of a small group were able to have spontaneous erections, but their erections improved when they also used Viagra®. A fourth of the group had no erectile capability at all. Other studies that cite somewhat higher percentages for potency retention note that this was possible with Viagra®. The nerve sparing technique and sural nerve grafting are discussed further in the surgery section in Chapter 8.

Is potency known immediately after surgery?

A patient's future level of potency is rarely known immediately after treatment. Any therapy is a shock to the system. After surgery, it may take two years (and sometimes longer) to recover and to find out how potent you really are, although some medical centers quote shorter times. This has been confirmed by several survivors, but most survivors tell us that no one ever told them this in advance. Rather than trust to chance, men may want to ask their urologists about penile rehabilitation therapy. This approach is initiated for surgery patients within three months after surgery and is described in more detail in Chapter 8.

Will my penis be shorter after radical prostatectomy surgery? If it is, can I still have intercourse?

The penis may be anywhere from one quarter of an inch to about one and half inches shorter. The main reasons are lack of use, less circulation, and scarring. Initiating a penile rehabilitation program as described in Chapter 8 may improve circulation and keep the penile tissue from atrophying. The length of the penis does not affect potency. An erection satisfactory for intercourse may be achieved naturally or with medication. Penis length may not be changed substantially with other therapies, such as radiation, seeds, or cryoablation.

Ladies: Although men know intellectually that you don't love them for their "size," they have a lot of anxiety related to this issue. As a couple goes through the difficult time after diagnosis and treatment, it's very important for you to keep telling the man why you love him and what you love about the relationship. Don't leave out what you love about the physical relationship—most of its quality is not related to his size anyway!

While size can be a visual stimulant for a woman, most women are much more affected by touch than by visual factors. A woman doesn't marry an "erection machine." She marries a man with whom she wants to spend her life because he is a great guy. Maybe a part of that is that he is a great lover. And he can still be a great lover, even without a giant erection! In fact, without any erection at all.

Do I need testosterone injections to increase my desire or treat my erection problems?

ED is associated with many conditions such as getting older and lifestyle. A number of studies have shown there is no relationship between total testosterone levels and ED, regardless of the severity of ED.

Does hormone treatment destroy desire and potency?

With complete hormonal blockade, desire and potency will be minimal. However, current research on monotherapy with non-steroidal antiandrogens such as flutamide and nilutamide show that some desire and potency may be retained in seventy to eighty percent of men.

Can sex stimulate cancer? Can I transmit cancer to my partner through sex?

A recent study reported that some patients decide not to pursue lovemaking because of concerns related to the disease itself. These concerns include a belief that sex will stimulate the cancer and possibly transmit the cancer to their partners. Both of these are absolutely false. There is no risk of passing the cancer to your partner.

Will my partner have any effects from my radiation treatment for prostate cancer during intercourse?

One study showed that there was no significant increase in the level of radiation in the home from men undergoing radiation treatment.

What are the effects of treatment for benign prostatic hyperplasia (BPH)?

Patients with benign prostatic hyperplasia (BPH), a noncancerous enlargement of the prostate with resulting bladder outflow obstruction and lower urinary tract symptoms, can receive a treatment called transurethral resection of the prostate (TURP). Although providing the highest likelihood of relief of both prostatic symptoms and urinary flow obstruction, surgical intervention for BPH with procedures such as TURP can have a significant impact on the patient's sexual function. Two main symptoms affect sexuality: The first is erectile dysfunction, with rates reported as high as fourteen percent. The second is retrograde ejaculation, which means that the ejaculate flows back into the body instead of flowing out of the penis. This affects sixty-eight percent of TURP patients.

General Questions and Answers about Impotence

Do I need an erection to have an orgasm?

An impotent man can have an orgasm. *An erection is not needed for an orgasm.* The facts are:

- Men without prostates do have orgasms and simulated ejaculations. Pelvic muscles contract, so that you feel as if you had an ejaculation. As we will discuss in Chapter 4, different sets of nerves are responsible for erections and orgasms, so it is possible to have an orgasm when the penis is limp.

  Without a prostate, these orgasms are usually not accompanied by ejaculate. Some men may have a small amount of fluid, but most men will have a "dry" orgasm. Nevertheless, the orgasm feels the same as with ejaculate. The issue is not the fluid, but the feeling.

- Even without an erection, men can have sensations and release during orgasm that are similar to men with an erection.
- Orchiectomy patients (those who have had their testes removed) can have orgasms. Even orchiectomy patients in their eighties have had "wet dreams." The key to having orgasms is that these men have known desire and experienced orgasms, thus proving again that sex is in the mind.

Can my partner have an orgasm if I don't have an erection?

Yes, yes, yes! A woman does not need penetration to have an orgasm. Men and women are anatomically fortunate because the organ that causes a woman's orgasm is on the outside. There are many ways for a woman to experience pleasure and to achieve an orgasm, even with a partner who has no erection at all. Stimulation of the clitoris can be accomplished by several means. An erection is not required. Chapter 5 discusses means of stimulating and bringing one's partner to orgasm even without an erection.

Does satisfaction require having an orgasm?

Many men believe that an orgasm is needed for a satisfying sexual experience. Most women know this is not true. Many men have never given themselves a chance to find this out. *An orgasm is a wonderful benefit but it does not have to be the goal of lovemaking.*

If one medication, such as Viagra®, does not work for me, will another one work?

The different results in clinical trials point up the fact that not all the participants will react the same to a particular medication. Clinical trial subjects are chosen to limit the number of variables that can affect the results of the trial. Even with tight selection criteria, the medication being tested will be successful only on some of the trial population. Each person's metabolism is different, as are each individual's general health, diet, and level of exercise. Each erection-inducing medication is chemically different. So there is a possibility that one drug will work on one person when another drug does not at all or only partially.

Talking with Your Partner

Key Points

✔ *The three key words for romantic and sexual health are communicate, communicate, communicate.*

✔ *Talking with your partner is a first step toward reviving intimacy.*

✔ *Sex is only as good as the quality of the relationship, and the quality of the relationship depends on the partners' communication.*

✔ *One partner must bring up the issues of impotence and alternative ways to please each other in a loving way that opens up communication. Entering into a conspiracy of silence is destructive to a relationship and isolates partners from each other.*

✔ *Don't assume you know what your partner wants: ask.*

✔ *Every couple occasionally has differences. Couples can handle these differences by having their own conflict resolution process.*

I have talked with him until I'm blue in the face and I get nowhere. He is hung up because he can't get an erection like in the old days.

I worked with him after surgery and he was depressed. Gradually, he recovered a lot of capability. Now, he won't come near me.

I go in the kitchen and put my arms around her and she pushes my hands away. "Don't start when you can't finish. You leave me frustrated."

Three couples in a logjam. To paraphrase an old TV show, there are many such stories. One survey showed that, "[S]even out of 10 people said someone in their relationship has trouble discussing intimacy. Not surprisingly, the majority said it was their partner who has the difficulty." How can they get past the block? Often, when one partner puts up a barrier, the other goes into a defensive mode. The result is that getting the partners to speak to each other is much more difficult. Then, even if they want to, they can't seem to get around it, make up, and get the talk channels open again. Disappointment, fear, anger, rejection, and regret all overlap and interact. These feelings and behaviors must be recognized and dealt with if the partners are to reestablish good communications and a healthy sex life.

One recent medical article positions erectile dysfunction in the context of the couple's relationship as follows:

Advances in pharmacological, mechanical, and surgical treatment for erectile dysfunction (ED) now allow erectile function to be re-established in most men who experience this problem. However, re-establishing erectile function and re-establishing a satisfying sexual interaction with a partner are totally different objectives, and when the latter is not met, the man may re-present with treatment failure or withdraw from treatment altogether. All non-talking therapies focus on the penis as the dysfunctional element, and all too often clinicians fail to appreciate that erectile dysfunction can result from problems in the patient's partner and/or difficulties in their relationship.

The erectile dysfunction may be caused or aggravated by cancer treatment, but it may also be brought on by other sexual problems in either the man or the woman, such as difficulty with arousal, lack of desire, or fear of intimacy. And erectile dysfunction can be the result of sexual dysfunction in the relationship. Relationship difficulties may lead to sexual dysfunction, which can in turn lead to the man having fear and anxiety over whether he will have an erection and his partner's reaction to his lovemaking ability.

Don't expect anything to work right for the first six months after surgery. Many of us are encouraged to expect that we will be normal. Where sexual function is concerned, that is rarely the case. But talking with your partner is a necessary first step to reviving intimacy at whatever level you are interested. The talking can cover many issues, from "do we become sexual?" to "what does that mean for each of us?" to "how do we do it?"

Talking is also necessary to work on the fear and anxiety each partner has in becoming sexual again. The man might have to deal with an overriding tension. What if he cannot get an erection? Will she become angry? Will she be disappointed? Perhaps more important, will she look at him as not being a "full man"? She may wonder, "Will he be okay?" "What will he want from me sexually?" "Has he changed?"

Misunderstandings are always possible, and they become even more likely when there are overriding pressures and concerns. If couples have difficulty talking about easy things, the likelihood is that they never talk about the sensitive subjects.

Elephants Bite

"We haven't made love in the eleven years, since I was treated for prostate cancer," said the man to the group sitting in a circle discussing their sexuality issues. Impotence and some stress incontinence embarrassed him the first time his wife approached him sexually after treatment, and they never tried again. They also never discuss sex. A woman in the group said:

We had the same problem. It was like we had a big thing between us and it was weighing us down. It was worse when we went into the bedroom. We tried to avoid being undressed in front of each other. We had to be careful not to say anything that would make either one of us think about sex. It was as if there was an elephant in the bedroom. We tried to ignore it. But it didn't work. The bedroom meant loving and sex. Going into the bedroom meant that elephant would be there reminding us that no matter what we did during the day, we had to come to terms with how to deal with sex and intimacy. Finally, I couldn't stand it any longer. I told him we must work on the problem. I love him too much to live without affection or loving.

Many couples affected by erectile dysfunction have the Elephant Syndrome: They don't talk about sex, but it is very much on their minds. Their "fixes" range from the Utah wife who won't let her husband touch her because he "can't follow through" to a "husband who regularly has a headache." Then there is the couple who sleep in separate rooms so they "can get a better night's sleep." The stories are many but the effect is the same: Their inability to speak about their true feelings leads to an absence of physical affection, which in turn separates the couple.

Much of the communication difficulty is caused by each partner's assuming he or she knows what the other person wants. A wonderful nonsexual illustration comes from an episode of Garrison Keillor's radio program, "Prairie Home Companion," about a rural couple who were going to spend thousands of dollars they could not afford to give their daughter a fancy wedding.

The husband, father of the bride, would rather do something else with the money. But he "knows" his wife would be upset, and, if the marriage did not work out, it will be because it was jinxed without having a real wedding celebration. So there is nothing to do but go ahead with the plans for a champagne and shrimp party (even though they and most of their friends do not like shrimp).

The mother has two jobs and wants to do the right thing for her daughter. She thinks the couple would be better off if she and her husband would just give their daughter and future son-in-law the money for the event and let the newlyweds spend it as they wished. But she "knows" that her husband really wants the big wedding or else people would say that he isn't a good provider.

Their daughter would prefer to have the money for a down payment on a house. But she figures it is really important to her parents that she have a big wedding. And she doesn't like shrimp either! Each thinks they know what the others want, but since they don't talk about it, nobody's needs are met.

Sometimes, it takes "getting beyond yourself," trying to understand the other party's perspective, and just "being there" to come to a good conclusion. For instance, on one sunny Sunday afternoon, a couple agreed to make love around two-thirty, and they agreed he would take a Viagra®. He took one of his hundred-milligram tablets. She made several phone calls, and all of a sudden it was past the agreed-upon time. Her last call was to a sick friend who asked her to call back in a half-hour.

He started getting annoyed. Couldn't she show more interest? Why did she have to make the calls? Intellectually he knew she had to. Nevertheless, his ego was sore. He said, in an unfriendly tone, "Why did you have to make the calls? And now you agreed to call her back in a half-hour."

"Well, we could make love now," she suggested.

"No," he said, "then you'll be thinking about the call while we're making love. And if we're not done, you'll be agonizing that she's waiting for your call."

"It's okay," she said, "so I'll call in an hour. We don't have to run on military time here."

"No," he said, "you've already promised."

The stage was set for a fight. He was feeling frustrated and somewhat angry. He thought that making love wasn't important to her. He didn't question her love for him, but her actions seemed to say making love was not that important. He decided to do something that would take his mind off the situation and started to work on a project that he had to get done anyway—but that would keep him in the same room with her, so she could come to him if she was interested.

She didn't understand what he was getting uptight about. They had all afternoon. She would get these calls out of the way, then they wouldn't be interrupted. She thought it would be nice to spend an afternoon making love. Too often, they made love after eleven P.M., when both were tired. Also, she had the pressure of getting up early to go to work.

After talking with her sick friend for a few minutes, she changed into something she knew would inspire her husband, came over to him, and kissed and caressed him. He quickly forgot his earlier anger, and they had a wonderful, long, sensuous lovemaking session.

After lying in bed and talking for a while, they got up for a postcoital dessert of strawberry rhubarb pie and tea. Could there be any better ending?

Why did this work? Why didn't they both go off and pout, but instead had a wonderful loving? First, even though each was a bit annoyed at the other, they acknowledged to themselves that there was a point to the partner's perspective. Second, he didn't run off sending a message to "leave me alone." Third, she handled her calls as quickly as possible and then showed him how interested she really was in lovemaking by taking the initiative. They each left the door open to the spouse, and that allowed them to reconnect.

The more stories we hear about couples reviving their intimacy, the more we realize that they use similar approaches. One partner takes the initiative to talk about his or her feelings. Sometimes the other partner listens. Sometimes, the other partner resists at first: "I don't want to talk about it." In the end, successful couples get through the situation; they talk, and they come to realize that even with his erectile dysfunction, both partners can be satisfied. Perhaps it isn't in the ways they might have had in the past, but each one can get the pleasure and affection he or she would like. So the successful couples have found ways to get rid of the elephant in the bedroom. They are able to revive their sexual connection. Their first step is to talk.

The woman who talked about the elephant in the bedroom brought the issue to a head by suddenly saying to her partner one day, "You know if we go into the bedroom like we are, the elephant will be there. He said, 'What elephant?'" Then she started talking. She hadn't planned it and, by not planning, did not get worked up and anxious.

They were able to talk and decide how to handle the problem.

Planning for Talking

Often it is difficult to take the first step. In Chapter 1, we talked about the "Steps to Successful, Satisfactory, Sensual Sex." The first step, the quality of the relationship, defines how well the partners work and play with each other. *Work* is anything they have to do to keep their household working, such as handling their respective responsibilities and taking care of the kids if there are any. *Play* consists of the things they do together such as entertaining guests, going on vacations, or just taking walks. At the heart of all their activities, whether together or separate, they will have discussed them and decided what is to be done and when, etc. How they talk and settle important things indicates whether they have a good relationship.

Even if partners have developed a good style for interacting with each other, when the subject is sex, they may have difficulties in talking about it. Deeply personal factors come into play such as ego, their feelings about their bodies, and satisfying basic emotional and physical needs.

Improving the Quality of the Relationship

Marital counselors and psychologists who work with couples generally follow a six-step approach, illustrated in Figure 3-1, to help couples get out of the rut. The last two steps may be repeated as often as the couple wants until the partners get to a point where they have achieved the desired result.

Figure 3-1

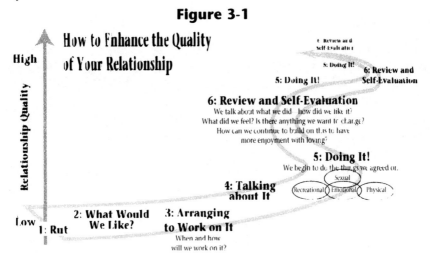

Step 1: Are you in a RUT?

The first step is accepting that you may be in a RUT relationship. A few or a lot of things are not as exciting as they had been. Many people would be reluctant even to tell anyone except in unusual circumstances that their relationship is less than they would like. Change is difficult unless they admit to themselves that they have a problem. This is very hard as well because it means accepting the fact that some wishes, dreams, and expectations are unfulfilled. Couples will have a breakthrough experience and take the first step to changing it—*if* they get to the point of realizing that their relationship aspirations will not be achieved unless they take necessary action. Perhaps the first step is just admitting that important areas of your relationship are not as you would like them to be.

Step 2: What would you like?

If you want to work through this on your own, the very critical next step is selecting the area or areas in which you want to work on your preliminary goals. To keep these goals realistic and relevant, you can begin with what you did before erectile dysfunction; this can be your starting point. For example, you may discuss how each of you sees your sex life as it is and what you would like it to be. Some people review their thoughts about the sex life they had. What is important is that both of you discover the areas in which you seem to agree that things are okay and, equally importantly, the ideas and activities you would like to be different.

Step 3: Make arrangements.

Key to being able to have a good conversation is to make sure that both of you will be ready to talk, will not be interrupted (e.g., not in front of the TV), and free from any other pressures (such as taking care of the children, walking the dog, paying the bills). Some couples have difficulties in finding the right time and place to talk—the "now is not the right time, I want to have a nice evening so I better not bring this up now" syndrome.

Decide where you want to talk. Some people will feel more comfortable if they do it on neutral territory, such as in a restaurant. Doing it at home may tempt one of you to jump up and get a cup of coffee when sensitive points are being discussed, interrupting the flow of the conversation. Then it is hard to get back on track. Or take the tack that couples with kids use when they want to revive their love life: spend a weekend at a hotel or some other getaway.

One woman kept asking her husband to read our first book. He never did. She decided to read it to him while he was on the treadmill. Since he was committed to the treadmill, he had to listen. She had his undivided attention. On different points, she would ask him what he thought. Gradually he started telling her his feelings. That led to what he would like. And he would ask her, "How do you feel about that?"

Here is the key to opening the door for conversation: You must set the time aside (even if it means making an appointment with one another) when you will do nothing else but sit and talk about this. You commit this time just as you would for anything you want to do or a meeting you have to go to.

Step 4: Have a heart-to-heart talk.

Now you are ready for the fourth step: talking. Your conversation will usually cover a number of topics.

The communication part will cover feelings, personal objectives, and intimacy. Intimacy is usually thought of in connection with loving and sex. But it also means closeness and understanding that can come about in other areas of activity, or *tracks* as we call them (intellectual, emotional, physical, and sexual). For example, you could talk about things you might do, such as read a book together, go to church, or enroll in a dance class. Physical and sexual intimacies are different. A physical track would include bike riding, whereas sexual may be anything from cuddling to intercourse.

Setting several ground rules usually helps. For example, each person should be permitted to talk without interruption. To avoid overlong, possibly rambling monologues, you may want to limit each person's statement to five minutes at a time. Although each person can talk about themselves, the desired end result should be an interactive discussion. Stay away from using "you" in the sense of "you did this" and "you made me feel like ... ." Phrases like "You made me feel ..." lay blame on the partner and can become the basis for arguments and disagreements.

When feelings are discussed, use "I" statements. No one can disagree that you have certain feelings. The use of "you" can have the effect of making the other person feel blamed and attacked, which ultimately shuts down communications. Each partner should talk about what he or she is afraid of and angry about, but both should do it in "I" statements (e.g., "I feel angry when I suggest sex and you want to finish reading the newspaper first").

Both persons have to be able to talk about what limits them and holds them back. A key topic should be a candid discussion of your body and body image. All too often, individuals' perceptions of how they look affect their views and participation in loving. In talking about deep issues and feelings, each person takes risks: the risks of feeling blamed, hurt, rejected, and contradicted. But these risks are balanced by the rewards: the chance to come together on mutual objectives and develop a better sex life, as well as a better relationship overall.

Talking about your feelings, hurts, and other personal subjects can be very intense and serious. This conversation can lead you to think, "I really don't want to talk about that." You may have to make talking fun. That will help lighten the atmosphere and make it easier to talk about difficult subjects. Some people find it helps to use board games, where, when a certain event happens, a subject is discussed or one of the players can talk.

Some people have difficulty in naming parts of the anatomy, such as "penis," and for others the use of slang words, such as "tits" for breasts, is objectionable. In some such cases, couples bought books about sexuality and read them aloud so that they can get used to saying the words. Alternatively, people take a piece of paper and write down words with which they are uncomfortable. The important thing to keep in mind is to reduce any reluctance that can make your conversation less effective. You want the end result of having refined your goals and decided which tracks to work on, when you will work on them, and where you will do it.

Step 5: Do it!

This step, along with the review step (next), will be repeated several times. Each time you do something, you will learn more about each other, which will bring you closer together. This bonding is the basis for improving the quality of the relationship and in turn setting the stage for better sex.

Engaging in the sexual activity is the act that the couple has been preparing for. This is when you try to bridge or close the gap that may have developed between you and your partner over time. Getting in tune with each other is getting to know how each one's tastes and thinking have changed in the course of married life. You can begin by doing things you used to enjoy, but doing *new* things may be more fun and interesting for both of you, besides breaking the routine. Different sexual and nonsexual activities will open the opportunity for fresh conversations because part of it will be based on the anticipation of new experiences. To begin developing physical intimacy, you might have scheduled time to go swimming, walk, have a barbecue for two, or even take a day trip to a museum. You might even decide to have one of you plan a surprise weekend trip.

For initial sexual activity you could engage in what is called *sensate focus,* essentially nonsexual massage in which the partners stay away from the genitals. Lack of sensate focus is considered the most common, but correctable problem that men have. The point of sensate exercises is to explore and enjoy your partner's body without the preoccupation with the genitals. These experiences will open you up to a better enjoyment of sex. Good sex is a whole-body experience, with all your senses involved. Many books, such as Dr. Richard F. Spark's *Sexual Health for Men: The Complete Guide,* describe sensate exercises. We also discuss more about sensual sex in Chapter 5.

Step 6: Review.

The next step is a review, self-evaluation, and progress check. You have taken and tried the initial steps. How did they feel? You and your partner must feel free to talk about what you like or do not like about your activity. After discussing your feelings, you may decide to reassess and change your goals. This should begin to help you understand what may be blocking you from achieving the desired effects.

When you go through these steps, you may discover that you need outside help. Certainly, there are many publications. Some couples feel they progress better with the assistance of a third person, such as a sex therapist, psychologist, or religious advisor.

Two Effective Approaches to Handling Differences

Unfortunately, many partners feel that the marriage status accords them rights that are not consistent with civility, reasonableness, and ironing out problems together. Ego, the "I'm right" syndrome, and mindsets seem to take over.

So what's the solution? Two approaches can work. The first is that, *when one partner opens fire, the other does not have to shoot back.* Sure, the other's comments can hurt. But think about the underlying value of the relationship and ask, "Is this worth getting upset about? I'm sure that when he or she calms down, we can talk about it." Then make sure to discuss it calmly later.

An example: A man asked his wife for advice and when she gave it, he got angry and blurted out, "You're stupid." His wife continued the conversation as if she did not hear him. About an hour later after he cooled down, she said, "I have to tell you a funny story. A man asks his wife for advice, and when she gives it to him, he says 'You're stupid.'" He realized how absurd his behavior had been and apologized. And they returned to the loving and caring relationship they usually shared. Why did this potentially explosive situation not escalate? She did not react to his heated remark with equal heat. She stayed calm and, when some time had elapsed, she was able to bring it up calmly, and he realized that he had been wrong and should not have behaved this way.

Another very useful approach is to *develop a conflict resolution procedure.* It's like having contract with a partner. As with legal agreements, the clauses are there when they may be needed. But the terms are agreed on when the outlook for the partnership is great, everyone sees high potential for the relationship, and neither party is emotionally caught up in any issue.

One couple has the agreement that, if anything happens to bother or trouble one of the partners, the other person has the right to say, "You seem to be upset. What's going on?" Another couple has a time limit during which they must resolve a problem. This couple says they have never been angry for more than four hours. Furthermore, they have promised each other never to go to sleep angry with the other.

Differences in the partners' likes and dislikes in loving can be very tricky and sometimes explosive. Your culture, upbringing, religion, and personalities dictate what you like and what you will accept. There will be differences between you and your partner regardless of how long the two of you have been together. These differences will remain there regardless of your joint efforts. They may be minimized, but they will still be there. You can describe many likely conflict situations and decide how you will handle them. But you can't forecast all of them.

The only way to avoid huge battles—big "mads"—and the cessation of loving is to work out a way of handling them. If both of you are aware of your respective differences, the best thing is to discuss them *before* you get to the loving activities. You can discuss whether or not to engage in certain behaviors, or how to modify them so that they can be accepted. There is no right or wrong answer or solution. It is purely a matter of how you react, what you want, how you please each other, and what you consider mutual satisfaction. This same approach can be applied to differences in other areas of life as well.

When opinions collide, they can quickly escalate a situation in which one person feels insulted, put upon, or treated unfairly—and the shouting match takes on a life of its own. Sensitive issues such as money and sex can easily provoke domestic wars. One partner has to resist the temptation to return the blasts and take the lead in restoring the balance to the discussion. And it should not always be up to the same partner. Conflict resolution is not about one-sided appeasement; it's about addressing issues in a way that is constructive for both partners.

Sex therapists say that sex is a thirteen-letter word: c-o-m-m-u-n-i-c-a-t-i-o-n. Good sex is all about good communication between the partners—understanding what each one wants and likes, what makes each of you tick, and how to work through conflicts.

Sex and the Single Man

A man we met at a survivor's group meeting told us: "I'm divorced and would like to get remarried. How do I build a new relationship since I have been treated for prostate cancer and am impotent?"

He decided not to date a woman even though he thought he could have a great relationship with her. Why? Because he figured his impotence would create a big problem between them. He never even gave the relationship a chance.

His story is not unique. Prostate cancer survivors who are not in a long-term relationship often have a very difficult time bringing up their disease, as well as any issues of impotence, with potential sex partners. Given the emotional and practical considerations, telling your potential partner is a big dilemma. It's hard enough to meet a compatible person of the opposite sex. Survivors face the additional challenge of letting go of the fears and inhibitions, and sharing experiences, needs, and desires. All too often, the worry that "If she finds out I'm impotent, she won't want to have anything to do with me" can become self-fulfilling. Should you broach the subject on the first date, the second, just before having a sexual encounter? One man let his new wife, with whom he had not had sex while they were dating, find out on their wedding night. (She was not pleased.)

The key guideline around the issue of impotence is to be truthful. One way of saying it might be: "I know it's awkward to talk about this before we even get to the point of an intimate relationship, but I feel I owe you the truth. I've told you about my cancer and the treatment. The treatment left me able to get only a partial erection. We can still have wonderful sex whether I have an erection or not—it will be a little different than it used to be." If the discussion progresses (and it won't always, we must admit that this may be a deal killer for some women), you can explain that there are aids that can help you attain and maintain an erection.

Reviving Loving

✔ *After years of togetherness, the emotional vibrancy that brought the partners together can get lost.*

✔ *Bring back the romance you had before marriage to revive the relationship.*

✔ *Creating a loving environment means paying attention to the little things.*

✔ *Relearning how to make love means taking time for talking, touching, loving.*

✔ *Make love when there is no time pressure.*

✔ *Make love early enough that you are both wide awake.*

✔ *Both partners need to know their own and their partners' anatomies.*

✔ *Focusing on the erection takes away from the pleasure of intimacy. Instead, focus on giving each other pleasure and showing your love.*

✔ *Each couple is different. Find out what makes both of you happy.*

✔ *Recovering desire demands understanding why desire has faded and working with the partner.*

✔ *Going to a sex therapist may be a good idea, and it does not have to be a long-term program.*

✔ *Creativity can enhance your sex life as well as increase desire. Simple ways to get started include changing the time and place you make love, as well as trying out new ideas.*

✔ *Expect that not everything you try will work. But finding new ways to make love that work is a delight and will make the loving more exciting.*

✔ *Just do it: Make love!*

We've looked at some facts about impotence and understand the importance of communication between partners. Now it's time to look at some practical steps a couple can take to revive their love life and set the stage for sensual sex—the kind of exciting and deeply satisfying sex that connects two people, which we will discuss in Chapter 5. The life cycle of a relationship follows a pattern that has lots of consequences for our sex life. Typically, the first stage is infatuation, characterized by excitement and newness. Within two to three years, the maturation of the relationship results in the benefits of stability and security. While this keeps the relationship vital, the excitement goes down a bit, and over the years routine and sometimes even boredom set in. We end up having "domestic sex"—uneventful, routine, and often unsatisfying. The relationship, the partner, and the sex are all taken for granted.

Over years the growing and nurturing things partners did early in their relationship may gradually disappear. So does a lot of the emotional vibrancy that brought them together and bound them. The Barbra Streisand–Neil Diamond song, "You Don't Bring Me Flowers," describes some of the symptoms:

You don't bring me flowers
You don't sing me love songs
You hardly talk to me anymore
When I come through the door at the end of the day ...

I remember when you couldn't wait to love me
Used to hate to leave me
Now after lovin' me late at night
When it's good for you, babe

And you're feelin' allright
When you just roll over and turn out the light ...
And you don't bring me flowers anymore

While these emotional developments take place, our bodies also change—inside and out—as we move from youth into the decades of middle and old age. We are not as easily aroused. Erections and vaginal lubrication don't come as easily. Many people find themselves in a RUT (Routine, Unappreciated, Tired) relationship.

If cancer hits, this compounds the problem. Slow erections become little or no erections. For someone who can accept sex only as the kind of lovemaking of a twenty-year-old with a new bride, this can be devastating.

But the sudden change brought on by cancer treatment can give a couple an opportunity to revive their love life and overcome behavior patterns that are contrary to those needed for a satisfying sex life. If a couple is reading this book, it shows that they have taken the first step. Instead of just accepting their sex life as it has evolved, cancer has awakened them to take a fresh look at what they can do to revive it. In reviving loving, a couple learns to express love in the many ways of physical intimacy. Racing to get to the finish line of intercourse, a couple can miss the pleasures on the way. In truth, getting there is not only half the fun; it can be most of the fun.

Relearning Loving

Relearning loving is about creating the right atmosphere in the relationship that stirs and increases the love-kindling emotions between two people. It is about gaining the knowledge and experience together that enables a couple to make wonderful love with or without erections.

Great lovers are made, not born. It *is* possible to learn how to make good love. Besides knowing the facts, such as the partner's anatomy, making love also requires an appreciation of the partner's feelings and the openness to using and enjoying all our senses in lovemaking. So how do you rekindle the fire—or, if you have it, make sure it does not go out? Familiarity can make for wonderful loving because you know each other's likes and dislikes, and the subject of improvement should be easier to talk about.

One woman told us that knowing each other so well helps her and her husband experiment and try new things in their lovemaking. The security of the relationship lets her "do things with her body" that she would not dare do with a new partner. She said she feels "free to explore new ideas." Prostate cancer therapy forced her and her husband to rethink how they make love and to share their thoughts and ideas.

She and her partner looked at their lovemaking as if they were creating a painting. Painters use brushes and paints to create an effect on a canvas. They have to know what will happen when a certain brush is used. The brush is the means by which painters create the effect with one or more colors. This couple thought of the "loving" brushes as the different kinds of kisses and different kinds of touch. A kiss on the neck might produce one effect. Running the tongue down the throat to the breast produced a different sensation. Together, they learned to use their mouths, tongues, hands, fingers, and different parts of the bodies to create a different beautiful experience every time they made love. This couple used their love of art as a way to think about their loving. It worked for them because both of them love art.

Another couple used dancing as a way to reconnect and to relearn loving together. You don't have to use an image like that, but it is fun to do it. Now when one couple goes to the museum and the other goes dancing, suddenly there is more hidden meaning in the painting or in the dance movement—a secret language that connects them as lovers. That is a powerful way to keep your love life vibrant.

The important thing is to find a way to reconnect that works for both of you. One approach to loving does not work for all men or all women, and what works for a person right now may change over time. People like variety. Preferences and sensitivities often change over time. After a long time together, it's okay to ask what the partner likes and doesn't like. Understanding what effect an action will produce in the partner is one of the key benefits of long-term relationships.

Most aids and medications that produce or enhance erections work only when the man is aroused. Pharmaceuticals do not create desire; they only help performance. As the expression goes, "When you're hot, you're hot, and when you're not, you're not." When you're not, many medications will not work at all, and others will not work as well. So before you resort to medication you may not need, you should learn how to get stimulated and passionate. The essence of relearning loving is regaining passion and rediscovering secrets to arousal.

Let's imagine a situation in which the frequency of having sex has declined over a number of years for many reasons. In addition, you have refrained from sex since your therapy because of erection problems. This has led to disappointment, embarrassment, and frustration. These concerns, coupled with a low frequency of having sex before therapy, have made it doubly difficult to recover the capability and the pleasure. Your partner, anxious not to upset you, retreats. She feels it is better not to push, hoping that, in time, you will begin to address the problem. Unfortunately, this is a self-defeating approach. The longer you don't make love, the easier it is to continue not loving and the more difficult it is to resume loving. One of you has to take the first step to get the communication going.

Relearning loving is a lot more than learning a new technique. It is a change in mindset. And it works best when both partners feel they live in a loving environment, not just when they get ready for sex.

Creating a Loving Environment

The objective of creating a loving environment is to make the relationship come alive again, to make it the vibrant kind of togetherness that you once had and treasured. Creating a loving environment can start with small behavior changes.

Many readers of this book have been married for a long time. For so many years, we focus on the kids, getting ahead at work, keeping up with the financial demands, to the point that there is very little time to think about what would make the partner happy. If we do think about the partner, it is at birthday or anniversary time.

The song, "Little Things Mean a Lot" by Kalen Kitty, is a wonderful prescription for creating a loving environment:

Blow me a kiss from across the room
Say I look nice when I'm not
Touch my hair as you pass my chair
Little things mean a lot

Give me your arm as we cross the street
Call me at six on the dot
A line a day when you're far away
Little things mean a lot

. . .

Give me your hand when I've lost my way
Give me your shoulder to cry on
Whether the day is bright or gray
Give me your heart to rely on

Send me the warmth of a secret smile
To show me you haven't forgot
For now and forever, that's always and ever
Honey, little things mean a lot

The way to remain interested in each other emotionally and physically is to show your appreciation for your partner in everyday life. A smile, a touch, a look that communicates "I love you" or "I desire you," speaking in a loving tone—they all build up the credits, the loving account, by showing that you appreciate your partner and do not take him or her for granted. Along the same lines, you can give your partner a quick unexpected kiss. When was the last time one of you went over to the other, put your arms around him or her, and said, "I love you" or "You're cute"? We like these little touches and the words. They help keep alive the feelings that we have for each other and don't want to lose.

TEN WAYS TO CREATE A LOVING ENVIRONMENT

1. Say "I love you" when you wake up or when you go to sleep at night, or do both.
2. Take an adult education class.
3. Learn a new language together.
4. Go to a movie or play, and have coffee afterward so you can talk about it.
5. Take a walk in the park.
6. See an exhibition at an art gallery or museum.
7. Read to each other in bed.
8. Do a crossword puzzle together.
9. Kiss at red traffic lights.
10. Give each other affection or love coupons or credits for something the other has done.

Increasing Desire

What do you do if one or both of you don't feel any desire? The answer depends on the cause for the lack of desire.

For men, one cause can be physical. Hormone treatment and orchiectomy (removal of the testicles) are the only prostate cancer treatments that physically depress desire. Cuddling, hugging, and touching are always possible and important means to keep a couple connected. The man's brain and nervous system retain the "memory" of what desire and sex feel like. So even though a man's desire may not be great while he is on hormone treatment or after he has had an orchiectomy, he can use many of the techniques, aids, and medications to fulfill his wife's desires.

Making love for the sake of the other person and the relationship is a deep expression of love. It just requires the man to get out of the mental state that he makes love in order to satisfy his desires and only when the muse strikes him. It means reaching out because and when your partner wants it. That also means the woman has to express her desire.

Another cause for the lack of desire after prostate cancer treatment is that the man is depressed over his inability to have an erection. Depression can suppress your sex drive, and fear of "failure" or rejection creates an anxiety that may convince the man that giving up sex is preferable to experiencing the consequences of rejection. This situation is a Catch-22 because antidepression medication frequently causes erectile dysfunction. You can look the monster in the eye and try to do something about your situation, or you can accept it passively (i.e., live with it), which means it won't get any better.

This is an opportunity for love and knowledge to overcome the depression. You have a chance to come out of the situation with a stronger relationship, a very satisfying sex life, and a deeper understanding of yourself and your sexuality if you understand that erections are not necessary for sex, and that you can have a fabulous sex life with minimal or no erections, and if you and your partner are willing to work together.

The first step is to decide that you are going to take action, and talk to your partner about your intentions. For the woman it's very important to encourage and support the idea, and be an active participant in the rebuilding of the sexual relationship.

A third cause could be problems in the relationship—a lack of the loving environment described earlier. To overcome this, partners must rebuild the emotional and physical bridges to each other, remembering that the nonsexual parts of the relationship carry over into the sexual part. We have an important maxim in our marriage: The relationship is more important than getting your way. It helps us to stay focused on the fact that the marriage consists of more than each one of us. The marriage makes us do things for the sake of the partner and the relationship that we wouldn't ordinarily do, and it prevents us from doing things that would be destructive for the relationship. (Well, most of the time, anyway. We *are* human!)

You should not expect your partner to be responsible for getting you aroused. Getting your desire back is *your* responsibility. Your partner can help, but there are also some things you can do by yourself. In his book, *Sex over 50*, Dr. Joel D. Block suggests, "if your libido is low, encourage and nurture your sexual fantasies. Read and watch erotica. Masturbate, but not to orgasm. Give yourself more sensuous treats, such as clothing that feels good against the skin."

It's normal for desire to fluctuate over time. Dr. David Schnarch makes the point that desire is complex in his book *Passionate Marriage: Love, Sex, and Intimacy in Emotionally Committed Relationships*. Desire must be looked at within the context of the marriage, with every part of the relationship affecting other parts of the marriage. Just as the marriage has high points and low points, desire will be affected and reflects these variations.

Every event generates change in a relationship, whether it is having children, going to school, starting a new job, going someplace new on vacation. Some changes are more dramatic than others. In their book, *Marriage in Motion: The Natural Ebb and Flow of Lasting Relationships*, Drs. Richard Schwartz and Jacqueline Olds stress the importance of recognizing the normalcy of ebb and flow in every relationship. By definition it is the pattern in a long-lasting relationship. "A couple must reconnect intimately through touching and conversation every few days or at least weeks in order to continue to feel close. ... Perhaps they had taken for granted that the relationship would take care of itself because their love was so strong."

Desire is essential in reviving loving. It includes wanting to be with your partner, to talk with your partner, to hold your partner, to please your partner, and to love your partner, in any way the two of you define love.

Pleasing a Woman

In a prostate cancer support group, a man shared the pain impotence had caused him. He said, "I want so much to please my wife, and now I can't. It is so frustrating!" We asked if he had asked his wife what would please her. He had not because he assumed that an erection was the only way to satisfy her. Once he asked the question, he was in for a pleasant surprise. There are many ways to give pleasure to a woman, and most of them have absolutely nothing to do with erections.

For men who do want to please their partner, Dr. Sandra Leiblum sums it up nicely in her article, "Women and Sex: What Do Women Really Want?": "For most women, orgasm and other physical genital responses, although important, are less related to sexual satisfaction than attention to the contextual, romantic, intimate and the sensual aspects of sex. These are the considerations that move women from adequate physiological function to genuine sexual pleasure."

How do you get your partner to this point? Dr. Leiblum identifies four major factors:

1. A loving context in which to enjoy physical intimacy, one in which they feel safe and valued.
2. A partner who is as much concerned about her sexual pleasure as his own.
3. Attention to the physical setting, including privacy, warmth, and comfort.
4. Sufficient sexual stimulation, both physical and mental, sexual, and sensual, with attention to touch, sounds, smells, and words.

To satisfy these four factors means that many other areas of a woman's life must be satisfied, far beyond the sexual part. A woman must be content with her nonsexual relationship, such as being appreciated for who she is. She must feel good about her emotional intimacy with the man, instead of continually being angry or for other reasons distanced from him in their everyday interactions. Women are not likely to get turned on and enjoy sex with them when they are generally not happy with their partners.

According to an article in the January 1998 issue of *Self* magazine, psychologists say that many spouses are reluctant to talk to their partners about what pleases them because they are "too vulnerable to rejection, too concerned that they'll cause discomfort in their partner and/or incur disapproval. For ... any of us, daring to reveal what we want sexually is to risk losing a relationship with that partner." They also say that, "Good long-term sex is not about manual dexterity but about eroticism. And ... eroticism is about revealing yourself and what turns you on—it requires a couple to be vulnerable." And to let themselves be vulnerable, partners must feel confident and comfortable with each other.

The foundation for the quality of sex is laid in the man's and woman's daily interactions, behavior, and how they treat each other. A woman cannot call her husband a "turkey" or a similar uncomplimentary name and expect him to feel good about her. Similarly, a man cannot treat his partner as a servant—"bring me this or that"—and expect her to feel like making love. When either or both partners use put-downs or other behavior that impacts the other person's self-esteem, it is hard to expect the physical intimacy and loving to be satisfactory for either one. The basis must be a loving climate, in which the partners live, and the things they share, so that they can move almost seamlessly from the daily chores to intimacy, loving, and sex.

Loving Is a Partnering Activity, Not a Solo Sport

Men and women have equal responsibility to make loving work. People born before the 1950s often look to the man to take total responsibility for the act and for the enjoyment of the woman. The culture of those born in the 1950s, 1960s, and later is much more in tune with the idea of sharing the responsibility (and the pleasure). But older couples often have to learn it deliberately.

The bridge for working with, being with, and loving someone is communication. Without it, you might as well try to make love to yourself. Communication may initially be difficult because men who experience erectile dysfunction are often depressed and generally find it difficult to talk about their inability to perform. Men do not generally admit they have erectile dysfunction. By the time they admit it, they have gone through a lot of emotional upset.

One of the great things about relearning loving is that you get to try new things and experiment together. If you talk to each other about relearning and are open to the new experiences that this will bring you as a couple, you will find that this sharing enriches your relationship tremendously. The communication will extend to other areas of your life and generally get you better in tune with each other.

By talking about it, you can become more sensitive and choose the most appropriate approach to your partner at any given time. The ingredients for stimulation depend on our psychological state of being at a given moment and on what else is going on in our lives. A person who has just gotten a big raise or the big job needs a different approach than one who may need comfort and support because of a personal downturn. In each instance, the incentives for physical activity will be different. Passionate loving in one instance may be replaced by the need for hugging and cuddling in another.

Learning about Your Own— and Your Partner's—Anatomy

We can learn a lot about our body and our partner's body from touching each other, sensing the pleasure points, and sharing our impressions with our partner. We talk a lot more about touching in Chapter 5.

Three different sets of nerves control arousal, erection, and orgasm. That is great news for people with erection problems: *Arousal is necessary for both erection and orgasm, but erection is not necessary for either arousal or orgasm.*

An erection occurs when the brain sends a signal down the spinal cord and through the nerves that sweep down into the pelvis. The arteries that carry blood into the penis receive a signal from the nervous system to expand. The nerves that allow a man to feel pleasure when he is touched run in a different path from the nerves that control blood flow.

Orgasms are controlled by a third set of nerves, which run higher up in a man's trunk. They are also controlled by the nerves that carry pleasure signals. These nerves cause the muscles around the penis to squeeze in rhythm and send messages of pleasure to the man's brain.

Thus, even if nerve damage or blocked arteries prevent a man from getting natural erections, he can almost always feel pleasure from being touched. He can also still reach orgasm.

After surgery or other prostate cancer therapies, sensitivity in the man's genital area is usually different. Before surgery, most of the genital area is sensitive to arousal. During surgery, radiation, and cryosurgery nerves are cut or otherwise damaged. A man may suddenly find that previous "pleasure points" don't work any more and that he has new points of sensitivity that he didn't even know or think about before. For example, after surgery some men feel a higher sense of arousal in the anal area than in the pubic area. This area was sensitive before treatment, but the sensitivity in the pubic area was usually so great that it overshadowed the response in the anal region. Similarly, the orgasm sensation may be felt in different areas. Therefore, you need to explore and find out what areas are sensitive and give you pleasure, and discuss it with your partner. Sometimes you need to "negotiate" a little since the partner may not enjoy touching you in a newly sensitive area.

Be Creative in Your Love Life

Being creative in love is extremely important for several reasons. Creativity leads to newness, which in turn produces interest, desire, attraction, and stimulation. Creativity can make up for a lot of difficulties and make a relationship exciting. It transforms routine lovemaking and leads to more desire and easier arousal. Creativity keeps the relationship interesting and lively. Many couples get to the point of treating sex as something they must do. Such a "chore" becomes dull and boring, as any job would.

Many people try to change the structure of their work, whether at home or at the office, to keep from being bored. Why not use the same approach where loving is concerned? It's up to you to make it new, to freshen it up. If sex has become boring, now is your chance to start fresh and liven it up by turning sex into loving. You can get ideas from articles, books, and videos, but don't underestimate yourself as a source of new ideas. Once you have opened your mind to the idea of trying new things, you will be surprised how many new variations on getting in the mood and making love you will come up with.

Peter and Julia, who decided to change their loving style in their sixties, told us they talk often now about how great and new it feels, and one would not know they have been together for so many years. Once when the kids were visiting, he pulled her behind the kitchen door and kissed her passionately. They liked it so well that now they play this game of "hiding" even when nobody is around. Barbara often collects a "toll" kiss when Ralph passes by. It's all part of creating an environment of permanent romance.

How about playing around in the kitchen while the two of you are making dinner? Or on the couch while watching TV or a video? Or how about going to a hotel overnight? The important thing is to get out of the rut where loving is done in the same place at the same time in the same way.

Why not dress up for loving? Being dressed differently is one way of introducing variety into lovemaking. We dress for playing tennis, swimming, and going to the theater. Presenting oneself as attractively as possible is a basic factor in mating. People do it by dressing and grooming. We did it while we dated. What's wrong with doing it now? Looking good also gives us more confidence in the bedroom as well as outside it.

It is okay to make love with things that stimulate you. There have probably always been clothes your partner wore that turned you on. If there's something special that you like, go out and buy it. Putting on a garter belt and stiletto heels may not be your cup of tea, but it's your responsibility to figure out what your cup of tea is and tell it (or show it) to your partner.

Making Things Romantic

There is also the environmental aspect: creating the romance. Use flowers, candles, music, or a little wine (only a little—too much will put you to sleep). Maybe there's a perfume that you like and that will appeal to your partner. Many people get excited by certain scents and smells.

Think of loving as something that you are going to do and prepare for. Thinking about it is one way of getting the juices flowing. When we were younger, guys would say, "I can't wait until I get my hands on her." They were daydreaming and imagining how great it would be. By the time the date happened, they could barely contain themselves. You can recreate this feeling with your partner if you let your creativity flow.

As you may know, some commercial medications require the man to take them in advance, and suggest that you should not get "stimulated" too soon, But there's nothing wrong with setting the right mood. It is also okay to prepare for loving without medication and much better for your focus on real lovemaking. It's a good idea not to take medication every time. This way, the erection becomes a special event and introduces variety into lovemaking.

Part of the romance is also what you do *after* the loving. Women of all ages complain that after lovemaking, their men just roll over and go to sleep. They would like the cuddling and holding to go on for a while.

Remember how it was when you were young lovers—or how it should have been! Lying completely relaxed after making love, talking about your relationship or the love you just made, where you got pleasure, or your dreams of the next time. You can re-create that feeling now, talking after loving. It's not a great idea to talk about money, the kids, or mundane things! This is your precious time together for sharing and intimate conversation, as if there were nothing else in the world.

Combine the cuddling after loving with a sweet appeal to her ears. Whisper in her ear how great it was and how much you love her. She will store those words away, and the next time you're in a romantic mood, repeat a few of those words, and it will trigger all these sweet memories and she'll just melt in your arms. The women should do their share of whispering too!

If you're still finding it hard to get out of the rut and recharge your love life by yourself, don't give up. It's okay to see a sex therapist. A therapist can work with you based on your specific situation. If you don't click with the first therapist, try another. If this area of your life is important to you, it's worth an investment of time and a little money.

Early Bird Special Sex

I don't understand it. In the morning, I can feel hot and want to make love. But in the evening, forget it. After dinner, I gradually run out of steam. By nine or ten P.M., I am ready for bed. In fact, I'm straining to stay awake until then. Unfortunately, my wife is completely the opposite. She's awake in the evening and not in the morning.

Human circadian rhythms, daily rhythms as opposed to monthly or seasonal cycles, show that we are not the same throughout the day. In any twenty-four-hour period, our bodily functions vary. These changes are reflected physiologically and biochemically. And they change as we progress through life.

This is significant where sex is concerned because most people make love shortly before going to bed. Perhaps we could enjoy sex more if we understood our body clock regarding wakefulness and sleep. The human body clock regulates sleep cycles among other bodily functions. As we get older, our body clocks shift backward. People in their twenties can go to sleep late at night or early morning and sleep until eleven A.M. or noon. As people grow older, their body clock shifts backward. Older people find that they are wide awake about six A.M. and ready to sleep by ten P.M. If you get sleepy at ten P.M., it's not a good idea to plan for loving at eleven P.M.

If you eat dinner at seven P.M. and follow the Viagra® protocol of taking the pill two hours after the meal and waiting another hour, you will begin making love just when you might be falling asleep. At that point, loving is not likely to be exciting for you or your partner.

Just as other parts of life change as we get older, the Lovin' Clock also changes. The recommendation is to have dinner and lovin' earlier. Both of you will be more awake and better able to handle the physical and emotional demands of sex. Making love in the morning or afternoon may add a whole new level of energy and excitement simply because you are both wide awake.

The Partner's Role

Successful loving after prostate cancer therapy requires both partners to be active. The partner plays a key role in rebuilding the man's confidence.

There are a number of key events in which the partner's reaction makes a critical difference to the future of the relationship. The woman's reaction may cause the man either to withdraw or to be encouraged. Sending a positive message can make a big difference in reestablishing the man's ego and in rebuilding the sexual foundation for the couple. Being supportive and loving is critical in these situations.

After a man has cancer treatment, the woman should show her desire by initiating sexual touching and lovemaking, and express her interest and support. She can help reduce the man's anxiety by showing and saying that she is interested in lovemaking, whether there is an erection or not. Saying that you're not that interested in sex won't help him much (unless it's the truth, and even then the partners should discuss how and how often they still want to do something). Telling him that you want to find ways to please him, along with sharing how he can please you, is also a good starting point. Reassuring him that he is still able to please you can make a big difference in the way he feels about himself.

- If there is no erection, tell him that an erection is not the most important thing to you. Show him what to do so your needs are met. This can mean bringing you to orgasm, or touching and holding you in a certain way—whatever it is you need to feel happy and satisfied. You can also suggest that you bring him to orgasm if he would like. We'll talk about ways to satisfy each other in Chapter 5.

- He can learn from you that it's not always necessary to have an orgasm to be satisfied. Encourage him to try it. Most men associate orgasmless sex with frustration. They will be in for a pleasant surprise if they let go of this goal orientation.

- If the man uses any aids that are supposed to produce an erection, you must both be aware that they might or might not work. You can try them a few times, but if they do not work, make it clear you realize that it is not his fault.

- Your reaction to his suggestion to make love is very important in the beginning. So what do you do when you're not up for it? Be honest. Tell him it's not a general lack of interest—just that you are very tired or not feeling well or whatever the real reason is—but that you really love to make love to him. Ask him for a raincheck for tomorrow or the weekend. Then you can reaffirm your interest by initiating loving the next day or weekend.

- Equally important is your reaction should he experience any incontinence during loving. More about these "leaks" in Chapter 5.

So you've tried to be the perfect supportive partner. But let's face it, you're human, and you slipped up. Your reaction got him upset. An apology is never too late. At the first opportunity, as soon as you realize that you did not say the right thing, you should correct the situation.

Here is what happened to Judy and how she handled it. Judy and Joe hadn't made love for five months, since before his cancer surgery. Finally one night he got up the nerve to start playing around, but found soon that nothing happened "down there." Judy realized that he was very upset about it, and out of a sense of protection told him that it was all right, that she didn't care that much about sex anyway. They both rolled over and pretended to go to sleep.

But Judy was kicking herself! She loved Joe very much and really wanted to have a physical relationship; she just didn't want to hurt him with demands. She figured out a way to start a conversation with Joe. It went something like this:

Honey, when we started to make love a few days ago, and you couldn't get an erection, I told you I didn't care much for sex any more. But that's not true at all. I just said it because I saw you were getting so upset, and I wanted you to stop hurting. Instead I think I hurt you more. What I should have told you is how I really feel: I want us to continue showing each other our love through lovemaking. We don't have to do it the same way we used to. If you don't have an erection, that's not the end of it. We'll find other ways to please each other. It's so important to me that we keep that connection. Can you forgive me for what I said? Are you willing to work with me on this?

You bet he was. He was so glad that she hadn't meant what she said that night!

Such a conversation can open the door again. The two words "I'm sorry" are very powerful! There are many times the man has reason to apologize too. For example, if he was expecting an erection and it did not happen, he might find a way to blame his partner. For some reason, it seems much harder to extract the two little words from a man than from a woman. What is it, guys, something genetic? If you mess up, please fess up: Women find you irresistible when you say you're sorry!

Take Time

We need time to make good love. Time pressure is an enemy. When we were younger and erections could be willed (and were sometimes involuntary), intercourse could happen at the drop of a hat. You will find that trying to get excited under pressure almost assures that you will not get aroused or that you will have a lot of difficulty doing so. Anxiety will hang over you. The more you worry about doing it in a certain amount of time, the more difficult it will be. So you do need the luxury of setting aside the time, then forgetting about time altogether. To enjoy making love, allow yourselves enough time to savor its pleasures.

Just Do It: Make Love

The key point of relearning loving is to do it whenever and wherever you can. Whenever you practice a new skill or technique in life or relearn something you used to do, you have to practice. It's true for lovemaking too. Not everything you try will work. Don't worry about it; maybe share a good laugh about something that didn't work—and then try something else. Practice makes perfect!

Making love is personal and individual. No two couples do it exactly the same. No two couples get exactly the same feelings from it, even if they do it approximately the same way. Everyone's physical responses are different. Just as all artists have to practice with different brushes, mixing colors, and applying them to get the desired result, if we want to improve our lovemaking, we have to try different things

However you want to practice it, making love enables partners to be connected. It counters atrophy of the penis. Make love as often as you both feel like it. Don't be afraid to damage anything. If anything hurts, just stop that particular activity.

5
Sensual Sex

✔ *Great sex is a whole-body experience—or, more precisely, a body, mind, and soul experience.*

✔ *Remember that your most important sexual organ is between the ears. Sexiness is at first mental; then it goes somewhere else.*

✔ *Both partners need to be aroused to have a good experience. Play to your partner's dominant sense (sight, sound, or touch) to heighten his or her arousal and enjoyment.*

✔ *Make it easier to get an erection by using positions in lovemaking that take advantage of gravity, thus helping blood flow into the penis.*

✔ *If you have partial erections, try partial penetration.*

✔ *Take turns pleasing each other. Loving means giving and receiving.*

✔ *Sensual touching is extremely arousing for most couples. Use touching to learn about each other's touchpoints for arousal. Touch each other for the sheer pleasure of it.*

✔ *Both partners can have orgasms without intercourse.*

✔ *Visualization and fantasy can enhance your sex life.*

✔ *Creative ideas and novelty are two keys to creating and maintaining self-renewing relationships.*

A Sensual Encounter

She woke up in the morning after he left for appointments. She knew that he'd be gone most of the day. When she got into the kitchen and went to turn on the coffee pot, there was a note saying it was ready for her. As she walked to the table to drink her coffee, she noticed the newspaper and an envelope. The note said, "I should be home by five. I made dinner reservations at our favorite place for five-thirty. By the way, you always look great in that blue dress. You know the one I like. Love you madly! B."

All day long she looked forward to the evening. It wasn't as if they didn't go out occasionally. And occasionally she would sleep in and Bill would set up the coffee. But somehow, his doing all this was getting her excited like a young girl. After thirty-five years of marriage, it was great to feel like this.

Since Bill had been treated for prostate cancer two years earlier, they had been having some difficulties. Bill was only fifty-eight, and the surgery had taken a lot out of him, mentally as well as physically. When he was diagnosed, he did not believe it. She knew he was in denial. Still young, playing tennis and golf, he was more vigorous than most men. She kept flipping between being frightened that she might lose him and being angry that such a thing could happen.

Bill came through the surgery well. He never had an incontinence problem. In spite of the nerve sparing surgery, however, their sex life had almost disappeared because he was impotent. But they worked on it. He tried an oral medication, which worked only some of the time. Injections worked all the time, but they did not want to rely on them. They even used a pump. With a variety of approaches, he was able to have an erection.

The hardest part was Bill's difficulty dealing with the fact that he could not have an erection spontaneously. He felt he was unable to please her. She kept reassuring him that wasn't true. With counseling he had gotten to the point of realizing that he could still have sex and that, most importantly, he was no less a man.

Over the previous few months, he had started spending more time playing with her, kissing her and touching her all over. Occasionally he would come into the kitchen and put his arms around her. Sometimes he would run his hand down her back and over her bottom. He seemed to find new pleasure in caressing her breasts, which she found stimulating. It made her feel desired and attractive. She had always wanted him to touch and kiss her more, but Bill had always been in a hurry to get to intercourse and orgasm. Now everything seemed different. Their sex life was more like she had always wanted it and thought it could be. They didn't just have sex; they really made love.

When Bill came home she was ready to go out. He told her she looked lovely. Bill had arranged for a corner table in the small restaurant and she sat catty-corner next to him. She knew he liked that best because they were close. As they talked, both of them felt as if they were in their own little world. Bill took her hand and she looked into his eyes and saw the love he felt for her. Sometimes, when Bill spoke, her mind would drift back to their early years when she felt there was nothing that could compare with the look in Bill's eyes when he looked at her. She couldn't resist placing her face close to his, hoping he would kiss her—and he did. They felt the magic of thirty-five years and began to feel tingly as they used to in the old days.

They expressed their love for each other and it seemed so different from the many times they said it in recent years. He told her how much her support had meant to him during the prostate cancer crisis. For him, that was behind him. He told her how good he felt when he awakened during the night after surgery and she was there reading. She told him that she loved him and that it was no more than he would do for her in the same situation. She reminded him of what he did only the year before when she had surgery. For the first time in years, it seemed, they talked nonstop. It seemed they could finish each other's sentences, even though much of what they talked about seemed new.

Suddenly, they realized it was almost eight o'clock and they had better things to do. She knew that after about ten o'clock they got tired and could not be as responsive to one another. In fact, some of the best sex they had in recent times was midday on weekends.

At home, Bill put on a record and they started dancing. She nestled in Bill's arms more than she danced. She loved Bill's hands gliding up and down her back. Bill started kissing her, and she responded passionately. Her entire day had been leading up to this. She had not felt this excited in a long time. Soon Bill slid the strap of her dress off one shoulder and gave her a love bite on the shoulder. She couldn't believe her feeling of arousal. Was it because Bill was going slowly or because she was anticipating what would come next? She loved her sensual feelings. She felt as if their love making was the only thing that mattered in that moment.

She was at the point where she wanted to discover Bill. She knew it always took longer for her to get aroused than Bill. She put her hands to his face and down his shoulders and back. He loved it when she did that; it made him feel like Hercules. She wanted to reach for his penis but did not want to rush it. With the way things were going, there would be plenty of time later. But she almost couldn't stand waiting.

It seemed like an eternity and yet felt so quick when Bill asked if she would like him to take an injection to help with his erection. She said, "This evening has been so special. We don't need it. Even if you come up partially or not at all, you can bring me around."

Bill started undressing her and touching her ever so slightly and varying his touch, more firmly at times. He began caressing her sensitive areas and she could feel the passion of the old days. Bill was not able to come up but it didn't matter. He brought her to orgasm with a soft penis. She then brought him around with her hand. Bill loved the pleasure of an orgasm by penile massage. Afterwards, Bill held her and kept kissing her after the loving until they fell asleep in each other's arms.

For her, the kind of sensual sex they now enjoyed was better than sex had ever been before. Sometimes she wished he had had the sensuality of today while he still had all of his capability before the surgery; but, given a choice, she would rather have today's sensuality than yesterday's erection capability. For Bill, their new way of lovemaking had opened up his world. It felt so intense. It was much more than a physical release. Experiencing all these new sensations and the emotional high gave him a deeper understanding of himself as a man and of his wife. It was also no small thing to see how much he could arouse her—after thirty-five years! To see her so interested and responsive increased his desire. And her letting him know how well he satisfied her sure didn't hurt his ego. Who would have thought that they would have fabulous sex in spite of—and because of—impotence.

What Sensual Sex Is All About

Great sex involves your whole body, your mind, and your soul. It uses and stimulates all your senses, taps into your creativity, gives you a feeling of being alive and vibrant, and connects you with your partner in a very deep and satisfying way. It feels so good you want to do it over and over again—and that's good because, the more you practice, the better you get!

Sensual sex is the way to have great sex after erectile dysfunction caused by treatment. One can look at sensual sex as being "time-released" sex; it feels good from the time you begin it, lasts for a long time, and feels good all over. You are enjoying every moment of it, not just the end. The "time-release" formula means that it becomes a complete mind–body experience. The creative part will allow each partner room to grow in loving by tapping into each one's loving potential. In sensual sex, arousal increases with the time and energy the partners devote to it. When you slow down, you can enjoy every moment of loving.

Getting in the Mood

The first of two conditions for getting in the mood is that both partners must be interested in and agree to making love. The second is to know how to arouse and how to become aroused. This is different for everyone. To cope and function as well as possible with impotence, it is important to know about arousal dynamics so you can focus on what has the best chance of working.

Women and men are different when it comes to arousal. Helen Fisher, known for her work in relationships and women, says that although men and women both have a strong sex drive, it differs between the sexes. Women's libido is triggered by different kinds of fantasies and different circumstances than are men's. Arousal is all about doing things that make a partner interested in making love. Certainly, a woman's arousal will arouse a man even more.

Aging and cancer therapy can contribute to compatible loving. As men get older, erections do not come easily or quickly. Focusing on performance is counterproductive. For a man with erectile dysfunction, an erection cannot be willed to occur. Erections happen only with positive stimuli that trigger enzymes and neurological responses, creating arousal.

Early in their lives, women are sexually receptive but do not achieve orgasm as quickly as men because women have a lot of estrogen, which tempers the effect of their testosterone. The high level of testosterone in young men gives them their sex drive and drives them to quick orgasms. As women grow older, their estrogen levels decrease so their testosterone has a greater effect, and they become aroused and achieve orgasm more readily. Men take longer to achieve orgasm and get more pleasure out of fore-play then they used to. By the time men and women are in their fifties and sixties, they are better matched sexually.

Generally, men tend to be more oriented toward the "sex" part (penetration) and women toward the "loving" part (touching and experiencing tenderness). But the two aren't really that far apart. Loving starts with caring and desire. Desire means saying "I want you" in so many ways. Both men and women want to get that message from their partner. What begins with tenderness, caress-ing, and kissing may evolve into sex, or may be cherished by itself. Sex without loving and tenderness is a mechanical act. One of the women we talked to told her husband, "I want you to come near me but not always to come."

Getting aroused is about getting into a mood, just as you would to paint, write, or play music. We're reminded of the time we saw Isaac Stern in a class of Japanese children who had studied the Suzuki method of playing the violin. After one girl played a piece for him in a kind of automatic, technical fashion, he asked her to think about the piece with her heart. He created the picture of a mood, a feeling. She played the piece again, this time with caring, sensitivity, and tenderness. The difference between her first and second versions is the same as the difference between sex as a mechanical act and true loving.

There is a strong interplay between a couple's relationship and their physiology. Physiology is affected when the relationship is bad or when either partner is insecure in physical intimacy. Sex therapists say that the presence of sex indicates a healthy relation-ship. Without sex, many couples are physically stressed, as measured by body chemical levels.

Part of arousal comes from a feeling of seduction and romance. Romance is a cocoon you can spin every day in your life. Dr.

Patricia Love defines "romance" as "an ongoing expression of love between two people." Although the "romantic love" stage ends in a few months or years for many couples, Dr. Love says, "romance can go on forever."

Many people think of romance as discrete acts, such as buying flowers or giving gifts. In fact, romance can show in conversation and the everyday things partners do for and with one another. A home life that partners see as filled with romance can mean that the partners are in an arousal-ready stage. It's a preloving phase. It just has to be lit. Many women become turned off—or are not interested in sex—because their partners don't romance them, court them, or really "make love" to them.

According to an 1873 quote in the *Oxford Universal Dictionary*, "Romance goes out of a man's head when the hair gets gray." What we know today is that romance is really not a matter of age; it just tends to fall by the wayside when partners get so used to each other that every aspect of the relationship becomes routine. Falling into a routine is like casting a spell on love. Nobody is interested in a mechanical act.

Sophia Loren was right on when she said, "After all, sexiness is all mental. It starts here [pointing to her head] and then goes somewhere else ... ."

So go ahead. Be romantic. Treat her like the woman you fell for.

• Make her feel desirable.
• Make her feel special.
• Say nice things to your lover, even if she knows you're stretching it.

Getting Prepared

Part of keeping the old magic going is to avoid turnoffs. Some of these actions may always have been part of your "routine." For example, showering and/or washing up completely before sex or going on an outing that could lead to sex. If you've eaten ethnic foods noted for garlic, onions, curries, or other strong ingredients, deal with that before getting close to each other. If the man's beard grows fast, he may want to shave so as not to rake bristles across tender skin.

Prostate cancer treatment necessitates some additional preparations. The man should void before activity begins. Prostate surgery survivors have only one sphincter and are likely to have a leak of urine during sex (stress incontinence). Have a hand towel or tissues close by, and don't hesitate to use them if necessary. Prompt use will avoid unpleasantness. It can be no more than a quick dab and will not interfere.

Let's face it, these annoyances will occur. The question is do you manage them or do you let them control you and interfere with the enjoyment that both of you can have?

Women also need specific preparations. As women get older, the vagina has less natural lubrication. In one study, about sixty percent of postmenopausal women reported discomfort during sexual intercourse, vaginal dryness, and other physical symptoms. It's a good idea to lubricate the vagina as well as the penis. KY Jelly and Astroglide are two of the better lubricants. Body heat tends to liquefy Astroglide, which also feels more natural. And then, of course, there is the most natural of all lubricants, saliva.

Other things some people like include perfumes or cologne, massage gels, erotic videos, sex toys, silky lingerie or other clothing, or silk sheets.

Sex toys include vibrators, rubber-nubbed massage mitts, simulated penises, and so on. They are available from sites on the Internet as well as from adult shops in any big city. If the partners are interested in videos, sex therapists and other practitioners often recommend those offered by the Sinclair Intimacy Institute (*intimacyinstitute.com*) in Chapel Hill, North Carolina, for instructional quality.

Of course, there is always sexy, silky lingerie. If a woman is too embarrassed to go into a store, she can order them from a catalog or on the Internet. Some people find various nonpornographic magazines have material that arouse them, such as the annual swimsuit issue of *Sports Illustrated* or even the Victoria's Secret catalogue.

Some people get what are known as coital headaches from intercourse. Sex causes blood pressure to build in many places, including your head. Viagra® has also been known to cause headaches. Taking a pain reliever before sex may eliminate the headache or at least reduce it.

Sensual Arousal

Most people know that their partners get turned on by different things than they do. Generally, it comes down to men becoming aroused by different stimuli than women. Without understanding the partner, sensual sex will be considerably diminished.

The way a lover looks, or a certain way he or she moves, can open the door to attraction and arousal. So can the feel of their skin. Touching goes beyond the erogenous zones; the texture of our lover's skin and even clothes can heighten our arousal. So can the taste of our lovers' lips, skin, and tongue, and the way they smell. There is a reason we sometimes inhale the smell of their clothes when they're not there. The right sound sets the mood—whether it is soft romantic music, rock, jazz, or Ravel's Bolero that inspires you—but the sweetest sound are the words of love and desire from our lover.

And there is the mental dimension. The mind makes sensual sex possible. It creates a whole from all the things we take in through our senses and adds more of its own, like the memories and the fantasies we create. Our mind gives us the ability to focus on our partner in a loving session.

Kissing

Very often, married couples get away from doing sensual kissing. The peck on the cheek or the quick touch on the mouth kind of kissing can be a way of avoiding intimacy. Deeply felt kissing will be sexual and sensual for most people. Kissing can be a wonderful stimulant for arousal and kissing throughout is a good way of maintaining a high level of excitement and connection. After orgasms, soft tender kisses are a good way of ending the sexual part and show each other your love.

Couples usually have one or two ways of kissing that turns them on: either by pressing the lips on the partner's lips or by touching the tongue against the partner's tongue. There are many variations on both types of kisses. Moistening the lips before kissing the partner creates a different sensation from kissing with dry lips. A soft touch of the lips feels different from pressing the lips strongly against the partner's lips. Tongue kissing is exciting because the tongue has so many nerves. A sensual lover may not only kiss the tip of the partner's tongue, but also explore many other ways to use his or her lips and tongue, from nibbling or licking the partner's lips to running his or her tongue around the lover's tongue, to exploring the lover's body with lips and tongue.

"Dr. Ruth" Westheimer writes in *New Woman* magazine (June 1994): "Kissing is so erotic because of the many nerve endings in the lips. Typically, women like kissing more than men, but there's no physiological reason for this. Many men simply feel pressured to rush into sex because they have an erection. Instead, if you both get used to slowing down, you'll enjoy kissing more."

Touching

What is the largest sexual part of the body? It's the skin.

Being touched is a primal experience. Believe it or not, one hormone has been identified as the touch hormone and is sometimes called the "cuddle chemical." It is called oxytocin and it promotes the desire to touch and be touched. In her chapter, The "Cuddle Chemical,"* Diane Ackerman writes about mothers secreting the chemical when they nurse their babies, making the "mother want to nuzzle and hug it." The same chemical encourages cuddling between lovers and increases pleasure during lovemaking. The hormone "... snowballs during sexual arousal—the more intense the arousal, the more oxytocin is produced. As arousal builds, oxytocin is thought to cause ... orgasm." Oxytocin levels are sky-high in women compared to men, but both men and women release oxytocin during orgasm, which improves the connectedness between partners.

Psychologists contend that oxytocin is the key chemical in long-lasting love. The body craves touch and quickly learns to crave the touch of one particular person. It's addictive.

As part of relearning loving, it is a good idea to have a touch session, to pretend that you've never made love before and are first learning about each other's bodies. The touch session is not necessarily sexual. You could start without touching the genitalia of either partner, and only in a later session include the genital area. In fact, creating a forbidden zone during one session can create

*In the book *The Art of Staying Together,* edited by Mark Robert Waldman (Tarcher-Feetnam, 1998).

more excitement, anticipation, and arousal for the session that opens up the forbidden zone.

Pleasurable touching between a woman and a man is always possible, regardless of the effects of cancer treatment. Touching is neither time-restricted nor time-constrained. It can be done any time, any place, for a second, a minute, or more. A touch on the hand or arm. A brief touch on the shoulders. It provides connectedness. It is on the path to the more intimate moments.

Carrying the touching a bit further, take a shower together and soap each other. Run your hand over your partner's skin and enjoy the way it feels. Use the opportunity to find areas that each of you like to have touched. You could even consider making showering part of the loving once in awhile. As part of the loving touch, one couple puts skin lotion on the one who has just showered. They do this as part of their everyday relationship. It doesn't usually lead to sex right then, but it sends the message that they enjoy touching each other.

Even if touch is not your partner's primary means of arousal, you can use touch to get there. In recent years, therapists have recommended touching and massage as a means for couples to begin intimacy and physical reconnection. Masters & Johnson say it well: "[F]or the man and woman who value each other as individuals and who want the satisfactions of a sustained relationship, it is important to avoid the fundamental error of believing touching is a means to an end. It is not. *Touch is an end in itself.* ... Touching is sensual pleasure, exploring the texture of skin. ..."

Feel the softness, allowing yourself to relax and enjoy the moment. When the man takes time to do this, the woman will feel free to do the same. Many men get turned on or simply want to feel desired when their partner caresses them. So do women. Touching, sucking, kissing, and even gentle love bites can be a turn-on. Enjoy these activities and forget about sex while you are doing it. A big part of sensual sex is to enjoy the moment and not rush for a goal. Savoring every moment enhances the pleasure.

Touchpoints

Touchpoints are areas of the body that partners may find sensitive and desirable to explore. You can kiss, caress softly and gently, and squeeze touchpoints. Some people get excited with hard squeezes, but many get turned off. The touch, like the kiss, has to fit the mood of the moment. That's why it is so important to communicate. Don't counteract all your stage setting and preparations by doing something that turns your partner off. Touching is a key to becoming aroused.

One magazine surveyed readers as to the parts of their anatomy that gave them the most sexual pleasure. As would be expected, the results showed that more women than men like their nipples touched and sucked (forty-five percent versus thirty-four percent). Both sexes derived pleasure equally from their neck, back, and shoulders being touched, kissed, and massaged. Twice as many men got sexual pleasure from their earlobes as women (thirteen percent versus six percent). A small percentage of both sexes reported about equal pleasure from their feet and hands. Your job is to communicate your personal pleasure points to your partner, and to ask about his or her pleasure points.

Touching can mean a range of things from running your fingers, hand, or mouth lightly across an area, to a light rub or massage, to firmer but light pressure. Whatever you do, it should be smooth and almost seamless. Some things to think about:

• Move around to different places at least every minute.
• Don't rub hard.
• Don't jump every few seconds from place to place.

At times the touching or gliding your hands from one place to another may be considered a massage. Focus on what you are doing, feel the pleasure of it, and sense whether your partner is getting the same pleasure.

With these guidelines in mind, here are some touchpoints. This list is not all-inclusive. Your partner may have other areas that she or he finds sensitive.

• Women may like men to touch or kiss them in the following places:

Face: Many women like a man to gently run his fingers across their face and to kiss their face and eyes. Touching the crown of her head or running your fingers through her hair can also be extremely erotic.

Neck: Gently kiss or touch the neck. The back of the neck at the base of the skull is very sensitive to light touches.

Hands: If you are sitting watching a movie or talking with one another, gently touching the back of her hand could help in relaxing her and getting her into the right mood. Stroking the palm has always been considered an invitation—and for good reason!

Earlobes: The earlobes are sensitive, probably because the blood flow is strong.

Feet: When she's resting with her feet on your lap, play with her toes or caress her legs.

Buttocks: Though not one of the most sensitive areas, many people find buttock touching to be a turn-on.

Breasts: The sides of the breasts are very sensitive because of the nerve endings there, many of which prompt women to become aroused. Some women like a man to run his finger or tongue from the side of the neck down to the middle of her chest between her breast or across the top of her breasts and down the side. Unfortunately, many men think that squeezing breasts hard will throw the partner into rapturous delight. Just imagine she was doing the same to your testicles, and you get an approximate idea about the level of enthusiasm this will generate in most women.

Nipples: You need to know your partner to know how much caressing of the nipples is desired. Some women find their nipple areas so sensitive that they are easily irritated. Yet other women find it one of the most sensitive and desirable areas that they like touched. Some women like it when the man runs his tongue around the nipple on the disc shaped, darkened area around the nipple (areola). The key point is that there are many nerve endings, and the woman needs to tell the man what is pleasurable and what is painful. Pinching and hard squeezing are usually off limits.

Shoulders: Kissing and even soft, tender, short love bites on the shoulders can get her aroused. While you do this, you can run your other hand across her back and lightly massage the area between her shoulder blades. Stress serves to tighten the back of the neck and knot muscles that lead down the shoulders and between the shoulder blades.

Genital area: Of course, the genital area, especially the clitoris, is very sensitive. The clitoris is the little "button" or "pea" at the top of the vaginal opening where the inner lips come together. The folds of the inner lips actually provide a sort of shield or hood covering for the clitoris. Generally it is tucked away and not felt until the woman is aroused. When it is engorged, it becomes larger and firm, emerging from under the covering. Running your fingers from the surrounding area to the pubic area and the thighs can increase arousal.

The whole body: There is nothing more seductive than the feeling that your lover wants to explore every inch of your body. Slow touching and caressing can be extremely arousing.

• Areas that men like touched include most of the areas that women do, and:

Head of the penis: The head is particularly sensitive. Stroking the side and across the top or bottom with the fingers or tongue also arouse a man. Avoid extensive rubbing of the very tip, which can irritate the penis, much as with the woman's nipple and clitoris.

Scrotum around the testes: The scrotum is very thin and extremely temperature-sensitive. Some men like it when the woman's fingers are cold and have been known to have their partner touch ice before they touch the scrotum. Caressing the scrotum can be very pleasurable for the woman and the man, but beware of squeezing. Squeezing the testes can turn the man into a contortionist.

Behind the penis almost between the legs (perineal area): Light touching and softly running a fingernail in the area will please many men. Check with your partner at the beginning.

Breasts: Most men have not experimented enough to know whether their breasts are sensitive. Many men are extremely sensitive to touching in the nipple area.

Chest: Many men like women to run their hands over their chests. It makes them feel manly and desirable, and it feeds their need to feel appreciated as a man.

Giving and Receiving

So often associated with massage, there is a giving and receiving guideline often suggested by therapists and others. This approach is often recommended for couples who want to revive their lovemaking and for couples who want to introduce variation into their love life. Basically, it consists of one partner doing something the other partner wants without any thought of receiving personal pleasure, although that may be the case. After the activity is completed, the partners change roles and do the same for the other partner.

Don't get frantic thinking that both partners must always be active at the same time. It's perfectly okay for one of you to lay back and enjoy while the other is doing all the touching. Later, or another time, you'll reverse roles. And don't forget that touching and being touched can give equal pleasure.

Penile Massage

Many men miss the pleasure of masturbation after they get married, perhaps because they feel that they shouldn't do it with their partner and do not ask their partners to do it. Since many women enjoy playing with the man's sexual organs, they can go further to help their partners achieve orgasm through penile massage. She can ask if he would like it or just surprise him by doing it.

Oral Sex

If you find oral sex an unacceptable practice, please skip this section.

For a couple trying to find ways to give pleasure to each other, oral sex offers a variation on lovemaking, a different way for having romantic pleasure, and when desired another approach to achieve an orgasm. Contrary to popular perception, there is quite a bit of interest in oral sex from older couples. The Kinsey Institute New Report on Sex reports on studies that say couples in their twenties are less likely to have oral sex than older couples.

Some people do not engage in oral sex because they think the genital area is dirty (more men believe this than women), because they do not know how to do it, or because they are concerned about what their partner will think. Some are afraid to ask because they might be asked to reciprocate, and they do not want their partner to know that they don't know how to do it. In the 1920s, a popular silent movie star was divorced because he forced his wife to satisfy his "unnatural desires." He was supposed to have said, "All married people do those kinds of things." Fast-forward to 1969, when Joan Terry Garrity, under the pen name "J," wrote how great oral sex was and described different techniques for bringing women to orgasm in her bestseller, *The Sensuous Woman.*

In one of our support group sessions, a woman described how she helped her husband heal and how they stayed connected physically: "You just kiss it until it gets well." Yes, she meant oral sex. Another couple experimented with oral sex and a vibrator, finding that both gave her better orgasms than penetration. The woman commented that her husband's skilled tongue is "a great gift to my pleasure." Notice she said "skilled." As usual, practice makes perfect.

Oral sex has been practiced for thousands of years, whether it is the woman performing the act on the man (fellatio) or the man on the woman (cunnilingus). Fellatio consists of the woman's sucking the man's penis or touching it with her tongue; cunnilingus, the man's licking and sucking on the lips of the vagina and the clitoris. There are many books that describe the basic techniques and variations of oral sex.

Three books that have fairly good discussions and description of basic and advanced oral sex techniques include Dr. Joel Block's 1999 book, *Sex Over 50*; the old standby, Dr. Alex Comfort's *The Joy of Sex*; and *Sensual Sex* by Beverly Engel (1999 Hunter House Publication). For those who will try it for the first time, here are two guidelines: (1) Don't use your teeth, only the tongue and lips. (Don't laugh— we've heard it all.) (2) Wash the genital and anal areas well.

Massage

Massage is an extremely effective way to tune back in to the sensual aspects of lovemaking. It is a means of rediscovering the physical side of your partner. Both of you are there—one receiving the attention of the other and delighting in the feelings and the other deriving pleasure from the sensation of touching the partner's skin.

For couples who have a hard time getting started again, therapists often recommend a type of massage that excludes the genital area in the beginning and just focuses on the sensation. It's called *sensate focus* massage. Originally conceived by Masters & Johnson as a two-week intensive program of daily sessions for the partners, current recommendations as to length and intensity depend on the therapist, the couple, and the problems they want to work through. This type of massage enlivens both partners. Both feel energy and sensations coursing through them. The receiver feels relaxed and cared for through the soft and firm pressure of the massage. The giver feels energy flowing through his hands from touching the partner's skin. Being in a situation when neither partner is even thinking about sex is a liberating experience. It enables both partners to experience and appreciate each other's sensuality. The key is that the partners must stay focused on what they are doing. Then over time, the genital area becomes a permitted area again.

Books and practitioners talk about several types of massages, such as nonsensual, erotic massage, and tantric. It is beyond the scope of this book to describe the various massage techniques. However, many videos and books do. Books such as *The Joy of Sex* and *More Joy of Sex*, and books that cover tantric loving also include much on massage. Dr. Richard F. Spark's book, *Sexual Health for Men: The Complete Guide*, and Beverly Engel's book, *Sensual Sex*, discuss sensate focus and provide exercises. Entering the keywords "sensate focus" on Google and other search engines will yield many sources of information and exercises.

Visualization and Sexual Fantasy

Visualization is a technique that works for people in many fields, from business presentations to sports. When used in connection with lovemaking, it can help a person work through situations to handle them better, improve technique, and improve self-image. People use fantasy to aid in becoming aroused, whereas visualization may be used to improve your self-image and general capability in making love.

Set aside twenty minutes when you are not likely to be disturbed. Some people find it worthwhile to tell their partners they are doing visualization. This shows the partner that you are really interested. Then imagine yourself and your partner in the most positive, loving, exciting, and mutually satisfying love-making. Or, if there were some rough spots the last time you made love, imagine how it could be handled better and what you could do if it happened again. If you think of any problems, these might be issues that you discuss beforehand. Discussing the problems will encourage your partner to tell you about concerns she or he may have. You might also try a joint visualization, a shared fantasy about being with each other.

Sexual fantasy is another way of introducing creativity in love-making. The purpose is to get the person aroused, and this stimulation can be preparation for making love. One significant study concluded that low sexual activity and low levels of sexual fantasy go together, whereas more sexual experience is connected to a greater range of sexual fantasy. Many people have fantasies of what they would like to have happen during sexual activity.

Just as in visualization, people can use sexual fantasies to figure out how to deal with awkward situations and work out ways of handling problems. Certainly, if you think you would like to try something new, you can fantasize about how you would like it to be and see whether there could be any discomfort and how to overcome the obstacles for mutual satisfaction.

There are a number of explicit fantasies that people think of and act out without difficulty. One is getting dressed provocatively for making love, going to dinner, and continuing in the mood that you've gotten into. Some people suggest that their partner put on a costume and they role-play, that is, act out the fantasy. Partners can do this when the relationship is good.

But the fantasy has to be acceptable to both partners. Any fantasy role won't come across too well unless both partners agree that they want to be in the play. You can start with something simple, like being at the shore and making love. For this scene, you and your partner can begin by wearing bathing suits and bathrobes or some other covering such as a beach jacket. Since water is known to boost sensual excitement, you can include showering or bathing together. Just make sure you limit the time in hot water such as in hot tubs or jacuzzi's, since high temperature can lower blood pressure and cause lightheadedness, which depresses arousal.

The limit is one's own imagination. Sexual fantasies are a good technique for getting aroused because you can introduce new images and things that can stimulate you and in turn stimulate your partner. People have images of where they would like to make love, what they would like their partner to do, or how they would like to recapture the feelings they had when they made love in the past.

Special Techniques to Assist in Sex with Impotence

There are a few things couples can do to improve intercourse or simulate intercourse when the male partner suffers from impotence. Some of these techniques focus on increasing blood flow to the penis; others on using the penis in a less than rigid condition to stimulate the woman.

Using gravity

Probably the best way for producing and maintaining an erection is for the man to be standing up. The man can stand at the side of the bed, with the woman lying on the bed. Usually, American bed height is sufficient for this type of intercourse. A pillow can be used to raise the woman's hips if necessary. This position can work for intercourse, partial penetration, and oral sex.

The second best body position that will help blood flow to the penis is making love on your knees or in the "missionary position" (the man on top). In the standing, kneeling, or missionary position, a man will retain an erection much longer than otherwise. Certainly, a man with erectile problems will not have as firm an erection when he is lying down.

Massaging the penis

A penis needs normal blood flow to stay alive. Nature provides for this through nocturnal erections, normally three to five times per night, which oxygenate the penis. If the penis does not get enough oxygen, collagen builds up, the resultant scarring damages the spongy tissue, and the penis loses elasticity making normal blood flow impossible.

If therapy for prostate cancer has damaged blood flow to the penis, the man must rely on manual stimulation to stimulate blood flow and prevent atrophy. Men should massage their penis frequently or have their partner do it if she is willing. Many people, remembering admonitions from their childhood, ask, "Is it really okay to do this?" The answer is, "Not only is it okay, it's recommended." This is truly a use-it-or-lose-it situation. Recently, urologists have begun recommending that their surgery patients use manual stimulation as soon as the catheter has been removed, several times daily if possible. For more on retaining penile capability, see "Penile Rehabilitation" in Chapter 8.

Partial penetration

Many men can have some degree of erection, which allows for partial penetration. Even if there is only some engorgement of the penis, it is probably "stuffable" or "mashable." Since the woman's clitoris is on the outside, women can get significant pleasure from partial penetration.

Female orgasms with a limp penis

Even if the man cannot have a strong erection, a flaccid or partially erect penis can be used to bring the woman to orgasm without intercourse. The man or the woman can rub the head of the penis across the clitoris, essentially simulating a vibrator motion. The penis can be moved slowly across the clitoris, pressed against it (just barely touching or more firmly), or held in position against the clitoris and the penile shaft moved up and down or sideways. It is necessary to make sure the area around the clitoris is moist, other-wise even the soft head of the penis may cause irritation.

Another way of using the penis to bring the woman to orgasm is for her to sit astride the man while he is lying in bed. The like-lihood is that the man will not have any erection. The woman can take the penis and rub it against her clitoris as she wants. Even though the man may not have an erection or just a partial erec-tion, he can still enjoy the feeling of the penis being rubbed across the clitoris.

For changing the woman's experience, the man can also use his finger or tongue to bring the woman to orgasm. Guidelines to avoid turning your partner off are to moisten the area around and on the clitoris, move your hand gently on the clitoris, gently part the outer lips of the vagina, carefully lift the hood over the clitoris, and apply only slight pressure. Move your finger gently up and down or from side to side, and adjust your movement based on the woman's reaction. The key word is "gently."

The Self-Renewing Relationship

Introducing creative ideas and novelty into the sexual aspects of a relationship is one of the ways of creating and maintaining a self-renewing relationship. Stable relationships are wonderful, but partners sometimes become entrenched in patterns of sexual behavior. Over time, many people become relaxed and secure with the predictability that comes from knowing the established patterns and their partner. While this is comfortable, it can also lead to relationship stagnation.

On the positive side, the maturing of a relationship provides a safe arena within which the partners can be creative, exploratory, and innovative, thereby continually renewing the relationship. Over the years the partners may have separately and jointly transitioned through stages such as education and parenting. They have also gone from infatuation and "hot and heavy love" into a well-founded relationship. Transitioning never stops. A relationship has movement and continuity. Partners can take advantage of these attributes and keep the relationship vibrant.

Realizing that not everything they will try will work, couples in self-renewing relationships are willing to accept risk because they know how exciting it is to discover new things together, and how the sense of introducing novelty into their lovemaking creates its own sense of exhilaration.

Getting into Shape for Sex

Key Points

✔ *Sex is strenuous. Being physically fit increases the probability of having better sex.*

✔ *Exercise and a good diet improve body image, self-confidence, and sexual appeal, all of which heighten desire and improve sex.*

✔ *Avoid fatty foods, which clog the arteries in the penis as well as in the rest of the body.*

✔ *Eating healthy for sex is eating healthy for life. Effective weight control includes managing sugar and fat intake.*

✔ *Staying in shape improves your physical life, including the sexual part.*

✔ *Burning two hundred calories in exercise daily can be done even in fifteen-minute sessions.*

✔ *Aerobic exercise like walking and swimming, along with strength training, are beneficial for sexual and general conditioning.*

✔ *Pelvic floor exercises may be a noninvasive, effective means for controlling venous leakage (blood flowing out of the penis, resulting in loss of the erection).*

We of the Charles Atlas generation can still visualize the ad showing the scrawny kid getting sand kicked in his face by a bully. The ad went on to say that if you use Atlas's dynamic tension, that won't happen to you. Atlas may have sold more kits if he had also said that you would also be physically fit for sex.

You don't have to look like Atlas to be physically fit for sex. But you do have to be physically fit to have great sex because sex takes a lot of energy. Unfortunately, more Americans today are overweight than ever before, and they spend too much time in front of the television instead of on the treadmill, in the swimming pool, or at the tennis court. The combination of poor diet, lack of exercise, and allowing a relationship to fall into routines can lead to disappointment. Add prostate cancer to this mix and many men feel there is no sense even trying to have sex.

If men knew that exercising, even in moderation, several times a week could mean better sex, they would probably do it. If they knew that eating right would mean better sex, they would probably do it. If they knew that regular exercise and better diet would mean better sex *and* reduce the probability of cancer recurrence, they would almost definitely do that. In August 2003 a group of scientists at the University of California at Los Angeles (UCLA) reported that the Pritikin Diet, along with a formal exercise program, killed prostate cancer cells. Diet and exercise can't be separated. Doing one without the other only tackles part of the problem. Dr. James Barnard, lead investigator in the UCLA study, said that, "Our research found that the Pritikin diet and exercise program is almost twice as effective as exercise alone for inducing apoptosis, or cell death, in prostate cancer cells."

The National Institute on Aging reports that two-thirds of older adults do not do regular physical activity. Such a sedentary lifestyle not only contributes to excessive weight, but also brings an additional set of potential health problems with it, such as heart disease and diabetes. (And guess what: Heart disease and diabetes can cause impotence too.) The good news is that lifestyle changes, consisting of diet modification and thirty minutes of daily exercise, can lead to significant improvements. For example, the Diabetes Prevention Program found that, "Lifestyle intervention worked as well in men and women and in all the ethnic groups. It also worked well in people age 60 and older, who have a nearly 20 percent prevalence of diabetes, reducing the development of diabetes by 71 percent."

One man who divorced in middle age found that his ongoing diet and exercise program gave him a body that looked twenty years younger. He said this was the reason he enjoyed and survived his second tour of singledom. It also contributed significantly to his love life. He felt good about himself, and his partners were equally interested.

Increased exercise has even been shown to be good for warding off mental deterioration that can occur as we age. Studies have show that as much as twenty percent of the oxygen taken in during exercise goes to the brain. One study reported in 2003 concluded that "exercise increases the chemicals in the brain that help brain cells communicate with each other. It also helps the brain grow new neurons in the region known as the hippocampus, which controls learning and memory." Another study showed that "exercise helps foster blood vessel development in the brain ... ."

Another benefit of exercise and an improved diet is a better body image. You don't need an Atlas-like body, with "six-pack abs," but neither should you have a case of Dunlop's disease, where the "spare tire" "done lop" over the belt buckle. One woman we know told her husband, "You know I love you the way you are, but that gut over hanging does not inspire me." A better looking body is usually a better feeling body. And the evidence seems pretty clear that diet and exercise can help you look better, feel better, and therefore feel better about yourself. In turn, feeling better (and better about yourself) can make you a more attractive person to a partner in either a long-term or a new relationship. And that can lead to a better sexual relationship.

Let's start with eating right, then discuss exercise in general, and finally describe the specific exercises men can use after prostate cancer treatment to improve potency.

Eating Right

According to the Centers for Disease Control and Prevention, about two-thirds of adult Americans are at least overweight and one-third are clinically obese. We're not nutritionists, so for specific information on portion sizes, recipes, etc., we'll provide references only.

Dr. Charles Myers, a world famous prostate cancer oncologist, publishes a monthly newsletter with nutritional information for prostate cancer patients and has co-authored a book with nutritional guidelines and recipes, *Eating Your Way to Better Health* (Rivanna Health Publications: Charlottesville, Virginia, 2000). The Administration on Aging (*www.aoa.gov*) and Prostate Cancer Foundation (formerly CaPCure, *www.prostatecancerfoundation.org*) also provide valuable nutrition advice.

Some basic facts are worth repeating. Fatty foods in general increase weight, and some research shows that they might promote the recurrence of prostate cancer. Fatty foods and red meats do create fatty deposits, which can clog the blood vessels in the penis. So for many men the choice is simple—steak or sex. Seriously, it's a good idea to cut down on red meat and all fats.

Many people try to reduce weight by cutting down or eliminating sweets. But this alone is not enough. Nutritionists and physiologists have determined that if the body cannot process sugar, it also has difficulty handling cholesterol, and vice versa. Although many people may appear to handle sugar (e.g., they do not have diabetes) even if their cholesterol is high, or the other way around, the fact that at least one of these indicators is high says that the body is not metabolizing either sugar or cholesterol as efficiently as possible. Excess weight may be another sign of the body's inability to cope with sugar and fats.

Exercising

So cutting down on sweets (candy, cookies, doughnuts, etc.) and fats (red meat, sour cream and butter on the potato, etc.) is a good place to start a weight reduction campaign, along with eating smaller portions and drinking lots of water. But it is not enough. You need to add an exercise component to the diet.

Exercise does a number of useful things. First, it takes your mind off the next meal (don't laugh).

Second, exercise helps your body use the calories you take in more efficiently. Remember, a calorie is a unit of measure (the energy it takes to raise one gram of water one degree centigrade). If you are burning fuel through exercise, you need more fuel than you do just sitting around; so if you exercise you may not have to reduce your daily caloric intake as much as you thought. Taking in "better" calories (those that your body can burn more efficiently) and actually burning them through exercise is the key not only to weight loss but to conditioning.

Sex is stressful on the body. A June 2003 medical journal article by Günter Görge evaluated the amount of energy expended during sex. As would be expected, "Cardiac and metabolic expenditures during sexual intercourse will vary depending on the type of sexual activity." When the man is on top, he will expend the same energy as if he were walking 3.3 miles to 5.0 miles per hour—essentially walking a twelve- to eighteen-minute mile.

After one prostate cancer support group meeting, a man asked us if we knew the "best exercises" for sex. We started listing them, when he interrupted by saying, "So if I do all this, what difference will it make?" He went on to say, "I'm kidding myself. For us, sex isn't very passionate. Oh, don't get me wrong. I get excited and so does my wife. But it's more of a calm excitement. We don't go thrashing around on the bed or the floor." Would he like it to be different, we asked him? "Oh, yes, but at my age, what else can I expect?"

I asked him whether he noticed if his heart rate went up and was breathing hard and fast. "Oh sure," he said, "doesn't every-one's?" I asked him whether he sometimes feels as if he is out of breath. "Oh, yes. Then we both roll over and go to sleep. I am too tired afterward to do anything else." Sometimes, he wonders whether he will have enough energy to finish. And he hadn't even realized that sex was a kind of exercise too.

A man can do a quick test to see if he is fit enough for good sex: Walk two miles. If it takes forty minutes (twenty minutes per mile), he's generating less cardiac stress than the researchers say he would experience during sex.

It's not just about being able to engage in sex; it's about wanting to engage in sex. Numerous studies have shown that physically active people are more receptive to sex, have greater sexual desire, and, most important, are better able to participate in sexual activity. A 1998 technical paper dealing with prostate cancer patients' quality of life showed that "sexual function correlated positively with physical vigor ... implying that impotence may have an effect on general HRQOL [health-related quality of life]."

As little as thirty minutes of aerobic exercise weekly can rejuvenate a man. An extreme example admittedly is the case of a sixty-year-old patient in a wheelchair with ever worsening neurological problems. Dr. John Blazina, a physiological neurologist, told him to do one hour of aerobic exercise daily. The patient complained saying, "Hey doc, don't you see I can't do anything. I am in a wheelchair." The neurologist said, "I can see that and I think you need aerobic exercise to get the blood flowing throughout your system." Six months later, the patient was walking fairly well and hardly needed his walker. He progressively improved. About seven years later when he was back in a wheelchair for other reasons, the doctor said he was sorry. The man said, "Are you crazy? Your advice gave me seven wonderful years. I would not have had them without doing the exercise."

Many experts in physical conditioning also extol the benefits of doing strength training. Since men with prostate cancer should be concerned about bone mineral density, strength or weight training is important. Miriam E. Nelson, of the Friedman School of Nutrition Science and Policy at Tufts University, notes that "Strength training also helps reduce the symptoms of various chronic diseases such as arthritis, depression, type 2 diabetes, osteoporosis, sleep disorders and heart disease and, when combined with balance training, reduces falls." Finally, an August 2003 clinical paper concluded that physical exercise was inversely associated with erectile dysfunction (ED). In other words, the more exercise you do, the less likely you are to have ED.

About a half-hour of a slow walk will burn a hundred calories. Dr. Irwin Goldstein, a prominent impotence expert, said that a man needs to burn two-hundred calories a day in exercise to reduce impotence. Another study, using a population of Harvard University health professionals and published in the *Annals of Internal Medicine,* found that "Men who exercise 3–5 hours a week have 30% less risk of having erectile dysfunction."

Physical Activity and Routines

At the beginning of a physical conditioning program, it is not necessary to be doing thirty minutes of exercise at one time. An easy way to begin is to work it into your daily activities (e.g., walk up the stairs instead of taking an elevator, rake leaves and mow the lawn instead of hiring the neighborhood teenager). Many shopping malls open early for people who want to do their walking inside. For weight training, lifting cans of food or shopping bags often enough begins to increase muscle mass and strength as well as bone mass.

Over time, a regular pattern (three to four times weekly) of walking, jogging, swimming, or cycling is the best form of aerobic activity. Strength exercises such as lifting weights or using tension machines can be done two to three times weekly on the nonaerobic days. A day off each week is not a luxury; for most nonfanatical exercisers, a day off makes the exercise feel less like a chore and more like a part of the normal week's activity.

If you want to exercise with other people, organizations and groups in most neighborhoods have programs that will fit your schedule and desired level of physical activity. One man goes to a small local gym where the strength and flexibility class consists of a number of twenty- and thirty-something women. He says that he feels good when he can do some things they do, and some exercises they can't do. One exercise using a nine-pound body bar was difficult for him two years ago. Today he uses an eighteen-pound bar. He says sex is much better in spite of his impotence problems. A recent news story highlighted the story of one couple who started exercising in 1975 at their local gym. Her daily abdominal exercise is four-hundred crunches (the current version of the sit-ups we did as kids.) Her husband does several hundred. He's ninety-two, she's eighty-six. They work out two hours daily.

Some people are quantitative types and like to measure what they are doing so that they can see they are making progress. If this is important for you, you can develop a simple chart to track the amount of time you walk or work out, the distance you walk, or the amount of weight you lift.

Three Web sites (*www.fpnotebook.com, www.cdc.gov,* and *www.walking.about.com*) have considerable exercise information. The latter has a Walk of Life Program some people might like to use.

The benefits of exercising are many and include a sense of well-being, not unlike the runner's high. This comes in large part from the endorphins that are generated during a workout. An interesting by-product of endorphins is that they also increase sexual desire. This is tied in with an increase in energy, feeling better in general, and feeling better about yourself and the way you look.

Add to this the additional stamina, physical flexibility, and capacity to engage in sex. If it sounds like you are preparing for your personal lovemaking Olympics, you are.

Pelvic floor exercises

Gynecologists have long recommended Kegel exercises for women to improve pelvic muscular control and to give them and their partners greater sexual pleasure. They are named after Dr. Arnold H. Kegel, an American gynecologist who developed his protocol in 1948 to help women control their incontinence after childbirth. Then doctors recommended that women who suffer stress incontinence do the exercises as well.

Over the years, urologists began recommending that men who have stress incontinence or leaking after prostate surgery also do them to improve continence. A Kaiser Permanente study showed that although two-thirds of the men who had at least temporary incontinence were "continent at 16 weeks," those who did the Kegel exercises regained control much sooner.

In recent years they have been more often referred to as pelvic floor muscle exercises. These muscles are said to get weak when there has been prostate surgery, continual straining to empty one's bowels as may be the case in constipation, being overweight, chronic coughing, and heavy lifting. Many organizations publish information and the exercises on the Internet, such as the Australian government *www.health.gov.au/acc/continence/info/ abfacts/pelvicmen.htm* and a British foundation site *www.continence-foundation. org.uk/docs/pelvmen.htm.*

For some time, urologists have been recommending Kegel, or pelvic floor muscle exercises (PFME), for erectile dysfunction as well. Anecdotal reports cite men who tout its value. In the past few years, several institutions and foreign governments have done much work using these exercises for continence control as well as in the treatment of erectile dysfunction. One British study reported in November 2003 that "pelvic floor exercises result in the same overall improvement rate seen in a large trial of men taking Viagra® ... found that 40% of these men regained normal function and 35.5% improved ... the study found that 65.5% of men with erectile dysfunction had a dribble of urine after urinating and that this embarrassing condition improved dramatically using pelvic floor muscle exercises."

While this study addresses the issue of blood inflow to achieve an erection, it is known that maintaining an erection requires high blood inflow and low outflow. The outflow problem is known as either venous outflow, venous occlusion, or venogenic impotence. In early 2003, a University of California urologist said that, "Kegel exercises have no efficacy in the treatment of erectile dysfunction (ED) caused by corporovenous occlusive disease... ." Yet, a few months later, a Belgian study reported that when patients were taught the exercises by physical therapists who also monitored that the patients were using the correct technique, "a pelvic-floor muscle program is a possible noninvasive alternative to treat patients with erectile dysfunction caused by venous occlusion." The researchers also noted that age was not a factor, nor were any other causes of impotence.

A German urologist and sports medicine doctor, Dr. Frank Sommer, conducted a study in which 124 men were enrolled to do either pelvic floor exercises, receive an oral PDE-5 inhibitor (like Viagra®, Levitra®, or Cialis®), or a placebo. The exercise had the highest success rate of eighty percent compared with seventy-four percent for the men who took the pill. His Web site (*www.men-and-health.info*) presents results of his studies and shows some of the exercises.

Given that responsible clinicians and researchers have conducted studies and reported on them in peer-reviewed journals, there seems to be some merit in considering PFME for addressing both sets of ED functional problems: arterial sufficiency and venous leakage. Since there is no known downside to doing these exercises, one could say it can't hurt to do them. However, it should be remembered that it will take discipline to continue doing them and, as with any fitness training, the results are seen over time. These studies talk in terms of three to four months.

We've heard the exercises described in a number of ways. Physical rehabilitation professionals recommend the following formula for doing the Kegel exercises. The nice thing about these exercises is that they can be done at any time, even when you are sitting in a boring meeting.

1. Tighten the muscles as if you wanted to stop the flow during urination. (These are the pubococcygeal muscles.)
2. Hold these muscles tight for a count of ten.

3. Then, while continuing to hold the above position, tighten the anal/rectal muscles. Hold both sets of muscles tight for an additional count of ten.

4. Do ten repetitions at least three times daily.

A similar exercise routine is also called *pelvic floor exercises*. The Australian government Web site has a fairly good description of these exercises, noting they are for incontinence.

In general, we see no downside because exercises will generally tone your body and, in turn, improve your lovemaking capability. Include exercises for your abdominal muscles, for your upper arm (triceps and biceps), and for your back. Back exercises, which usually include abdominal routines, also include back extensions and push-ups.

7
Talking with Your Doctor

Key Points

✔ Make an appointment and tell the doctor in advance that you need counsel regarding sexual dysfunction.

✔ Prepare for the visit by planning with your partner and writing down your questions.

✔ Rehearse questions so you know that you will have enough time.

✔ When you are prepared and know what you want, you will not be intimidated.

To paraphrase the title of a popular book, doctors are from Venus and patients are from Mars. Both must somehow navigate a big void in order to communicate effectively. Statistics show that eighty percent of men with erectile dysfunction do not seek help or talk with their doctor about their sexual problems. Many men feel that doctors are either uninterested in and/or uncomfortable with the topic, or that they are incapable of providing any guidance.

Nevertheless, for patients who want their doctor's assistance, several issues need to be discussed. It is important to understand the doctor's situation and plan for your visit.

Understanding the Doctor's Situation

Primary care doctors who see adult patients (either internal medicine or family practice specialists) are being squeezed by reduced reimbursements from insurance providers, greater patient load because fewer new doctors enter primary care, and patient populations who are becoming older and include more individuals with chronic illnesses that must be managed. A study published in 2003 in *The American Journal of Public Health* estimated that a busy family practitioner or internist would need to add four hours per day of direct patient care to provide all the necessary preventative medicine to his or her daily patient load. Urgent matters take precedent over prevention and handholding, the authors state. As a result, patients often feel rushed through. Nurses or medical assistants generally conduct the patient medical history interview, which includes a section about the patient's chief complaint. Then the doctor comes in to review the notes from the interview, conduct a physical examination if necessary, and discuss the complaint in detail. The doctor often spends less than ten minutes with a patient.

Patients often gripe that the doctor comes to a conclusion before he or she has heard the patient's story. Some research has suggested that a patient has about 27.5 seconds to explain his or her complaint, talk about symptoms, and express concerns before the doctor starts thinking about a diagnosis. Medical schools and teaching hospitals are today incorporating such criticisms into medical education, teaching students and residents to be better listeners. But most patients still visit doctors in private community practices, and it will be a generation before today's students and residents are firmly embedded in such community practices and seeing large groups of older adult patients.

Patients, especially those over sixty, learned as children to respect authority and power. Doctors, with their white coats and M.D. degrees, represent both authority figures and power; many older patients are reluctant to disagree with or challenge them, despite the push for us all to become better medical consumers, and ask for explanations. Given the time constraints on the typical patient visit and the learned behavior to accept what doctors tell us, many older patients leave the doctor's office unsatisfied, with only some of the information they need—less of the information they would like to have.

An article on the subject of being a better consumer of health care, in the Walter Read Army Medical Center newsletter *USToo!* suggests to patients to prepare for a doctor visit. "Be prepared, bring notes, bring a spokesperson if necessary, avoid ambiguity, have questions ready, but *most of all*—BE READY."

Preparing for a Visit to Discuss Sexual Dysfunction Issues

When going to see a doctor about erectile dysfunction, both partners need to plan the visit and agree on the objective of the visit and the questions they want answered.

Writing down your questions

If you have decided to discuss your concerns or problems with a doctor, prepare to cover all the points you can think of. Talk with your partner and write down all these points. Don't trust that you will remember all the questions, because you will inevitably get caught up in the discussion.

Once you and your partner have decided the topics you want to discuss, write them down in the form of questions. Both partners should have a copy of this question list during the consultation. One of you can jot down answers, and review and modify the questions during the discussion if partial answers to some questions are provided in the course of answering other questions.

Follow-up questions can seek clarification and more complete answers.

Remember, there are no stupid questions.

When creating your list of questions and discussion points, think of the following issues:

1. *What kind of advice and information do you want from the meeting?* Are you looking for counseling on resolving differences between the partners regarding sex, such as differences of opinion on some aspect of sex? Or are you looking for some help on a medical problem, such as erectile dysfunction, that impedes the sexual relationship.

2. *What outcome do you want from the meeting?* Are you looking for a treatment for a medical problem or for guidance regarding your sexual function? Are you looking for a treatment plan, a follow-up meeting, or for a referral to another specialist? The partners need to be clear on what they want before they go further.

3. *What type of doctor or other professional is best able to answer your questions and discuss your problem?* Which health care professional would be best for you? The choices are many: a primary care doctor, a urologist, a urologist who specializes in erectile dysfunction and other male sexuality issues, an ob/gyn, a psychiatrist, a psychologist, a psychiatric social worker, a sex therapist, a marriage counselor, or even a clergy person. Each of these professionals will discuss your sex problems from a different perspective. If you are concerned with how to discuss the new sexual situation with your partner or how to revive the intimacy, a psychologist who specializes in counseling couples on intimacy, a marriage counselor, or a sex therapist may be the person to start with. If your questions deal with the medical aspects of resuming sex, then a urologist for the male partner or an ob/gyn for the female partner would be appropriate.

It is important to remember where you start may not be where you end your quest for relief from a sexual problem. An erectile problem may be physical, in which case a urologist—especially one who specializes in sexual dysfunction—might be the place to start. But exploration of the issue might find that the dysfunction is not physical, but rather related to anxiety, and the urologist may refer you to a psychologist or sex therapist. Often, talking to the partners' primary care doctor, whom both partners know and trust, is the best place to start since he or she knows the history and may hone in quickly on the root cause of the distress and make the best referral for a particular couple.

Whatever the decision about where to start and how far to take the issue through professional assistance, the decision must be mutual. Unless both partners agree on the therapeutic approach, one person may reject the recommendations.

4. *Do both partners want to go to meet with the professional? Do they want to go separately? Will each party see a different professional, or will one person go and tell the other one what went on?* Generally, both partners should go at least to an initial meeting. Under certain circumstances, the partners may want to make separate appointments and then be together for a joint session. This is particularly true if you are thinking of going to a sex therapist or psychologist. The danger in one partner going and reporting the results of the discussion is that the other partner may well say something like, "Oh, that can't be right. You didn't hear the doctor correctly," especially if there was some disagreement before the visit. Since intimacy involves both of you, going together would avoid such misunderstandings.

Making the appointment

When you and the doctor both know what you want to accomplish, you have set the stage for a constructive meeting. The best way to make sure you and the doctor both have the same agenda is to make a separate appointment to discuss the issue. This appointment should be made face to face with the doctor, usually as a "goodbye" discussion when you are at the doctor's office for another reason, such as for a routine checkup. Ask the doctor whether he or she is comfortable assisting you and your partner with this matter (many doctors will discuss only sexual topics after the patient asks questions). If the doctor agrees to meet with you, ask how much time the session will take so that you can schedule the right amount of time with the receptionist.

For any of a number of reasons, the doctor may refer you to someone else immediately. In addition, remember that such a consultation may not be covered by any medical insurance you have, especially if it is not linked to an actual diagnosis.

If you are not going to be in the doctor's office in the near future and feel you must deal with the issue soon, call the office and ask if the doctor is available to discuss a personal matter or if the doctor can return your call. Ask the receptionist when the call is likely to be returned so that you can be available or provide the receptionist with a reasonable window of time (say, two hours), when you know you will be available to take a return call.

You should also have the office fax number and the doctor's email address. If you do not hear from the office or the doctor, send a fax or an email stating that you need to talk about making an appointment for a personal matter. If you do not get a response in a reasonable time, you may consider seeing someone else.

Getting the Most from the Meeting

A friend of ours who went to journalism school has said that the most important thing he learned there was that, once a subject agreed to an interview, the reporter "owned the meeting." This is true for patients as well, especially if the patient has prearranged the meeting and prepared the doctor for the topic at hand, made arrangements with the receptionist to block out the appropriate amount of time, and spent time with his or her partner to prepare questions.

You own the meeting, so take control, maintain control, and make sure you get from the meeting what you came to get.

• If the meeting starts late, make sure you get the full amount of time you blocked out; don't let the doctor shorten your meeting in an effort to get back on schedule, if you feel you need the time.

• Set the tone for your meeting by having your questions prepared and written. Your preparation will make the doctor realize that you know what you want to get out of the meeting and will be less concerned that the discussion will ramble off track.

- Don't be intimidated into not asking your questions. There are no stupid questions, only people who stupidly don't ask questions they need and deserve answers to. In the presence of a doctor in a white coat or a therapist sitting behind a desk, people often second-guess themselves and fear that they will annoy the medical professional with yet another question. Don't get caught up in that fear.

- Don't worry about taking too much of his or her "valuable" time. A professional will let you know when he or she needs to move on to the next appointment. If you need more time, you can schedule another session or get referred to someone with whom you can spend more time and more useful time.

- If the doctor or other professional uses technical or specialized terms and you do not understand, ask that the terms be explained better. Too often, patients nod and say they understand when they don't because they are nervous about taking up the professional's time or appearing stupid because they do not understand. Asking for more detailed information and for explanations should be routine, and it can be done in a good-natured, pleasant, and cooperative manner. You can use such phrases as, "Help me understand ..." or "What exactly do you mean when you say ... ?"

- Bring materials with you, regardless of the type of professional with whom you are meeting. These materials might include your medical history, as well as a list of all the medications and supplements you and your partner are taking. Many pharmaceuticals and/or supplements interact with each other in ways that you may not know but that an expert might have insight into. If any doctor suggests a new prescription, ask the purpose of the drug, possible side effects, possible interactions with other drugs, and how to deal with any adverse effects. Make sure you understand the conditions for taking the medication, such as the time of day, whether the medication is taken with, before or after meals, and what you should do if you miss a dose. Write down the answers to these questions, since this is usually much more information than the pharmacy label will contain.

- Bring a tape recorder if this will help you. If the discussion is rich and helpful, you may want to listen to it again to make sure you caught all the points, to clarify how you remember the discussion going or any particular guidance you received, and to adjust for any differences in your memory and that of your partner. When making the appointment, tell the doctor that you would like to record the session so that you won't miss any points or misunderstand the information. Most practitioners will agree to this. If your doctor objects to a tape recording, try to find out why and work to come up with a satisfactory compromise. At the least, one partner should be prepared to take good notes.

How to Be Sure the Doctor or
Other Professional Is Truly Listening

A medical or counseling professional who is engaged in the conversation will ask you to explain your questions or comments and fully answer your questions in return. The professional who starts thumbing through other papers, looking at the clock, or making sharp and abrupt comments is not fully engaged.

One reason the professional may not be fully engaged is that you have wandered off the primary topic and gotten onto other subjects. You must stay focused on your objective.

Use your list of questions to keep yourself on track, and stay within the time you and the professional have agreed to for the meeting. The professional's comments and responses may prompt additional questions. Again, if there is not enough time to deal with the whole discussion, make another appointment or seek a referral to someone who has more time for you to talk through all the issues you need to explore.

Commercial Therapies and Medications

8

Key Points

✔ *When using commercial therapies, remember that there are many different types of therapies and aids for erectile dysfunction, but no single therapy is effective for everyone.*

✔ *Consultation with a doctor must be part of the decision to use any type of erectile dysfunction therapy and to determine the dosage. Internet "doctors" do not count!*

✔ *Partner should be included in the discussion with the doctor and the decision about treatment.*

✔ *For injections, the doctor must train you and observe you while you use the technique, addressing possible complications.*

✔ *Each aid has its own advantages and drawbacks and problems, and it may not work for you. Don't get frustrated if something does not work; try something else. It's also very important for the partner to have realistic expectations in case a medication does not work.*

✔ *If possible, start with a low dosage and work your way up as necessary. This puts less burden on your system. Follow your physician's advice concerning drugs and dosages. If you have doubts about the doctor's advice, consult another doctor.*

✔ *Have realistic expectations. Don't believe all the advertising hype.*

For therapies and medications to be effective, the couple must create the best possible physical, physiological, and mental environment for lovemaking, as discussed in previous chapters. Commercial therapies and medications for erectile dysfunction can, at best, complement the work the couple does to revive their loving. Quite often a medication is an optional supplement that can help make some lovings a little more special.

The ED treatments discussed in this chapter cover the spectrum from oral medications to mechanical support devices to injections. Some new research directions are innovative and prompt great expectations for future treatments.

This chapter presents in some detail the major commercial ED treatments available today, and describes in less detail some medications that can be expected fairly soon, as well as embryonic investigations that might bring promising treatments in five to ten years. Certainly, if you know of others that should be included in future editions of this book, please use the contact information in the front of the book to let us know about them.

An important note: Sexual intercourse is physical exercise! For those of you who skipped Chapter 6, it is important to be aware that if you are not able to walk briskly (defined as a rate of at least three to five miles per hour) for an hour due to a heart condition, then you should be *extremely* cautious before attempting to have sex.

Is There a One-Size-Fits-All Treatment?

Ideally, it would be nice to have one therapy for erectile dysfunction. One article notes five characteristics required for a comprehensive, universal treatment. A one-size-fits-all treatment would be:

• Effective.
• Useful immediately when needed.
• Free of toxicity and side effects.
• Easy to use in the form of pills or cream.
• Affordable.

Unfortunately, this ideal therapy does not yet exist. Vacuum therapy systems and penile implants generally work well all of the time. Every available medication seems to aid some men at least some of the time. However, they do not work on all men. When they do work, they may not be consistently effective. Most medications and therapies work soon after being taken (they increase performance soon after being used, within ten minutes to one hour). Some new oral medications will shrink the waiting time and last much longer. Although some are easy to use, systemic oral medications have side effects.

When considering cost, it is important to separate initial cost versus per-use cost. For example, a vacuum device may cost up to five hundred dollars initially but nothing thereafter, whereas an oral medication may cost nine to thirteen dollars per pill. Amortizing the pump over fifty uses comes to a ten-dollar per-use cost.

Treatments: What Works for You?

A 1996 article by Dr. Jonathan P. Jarow assessed patient preference and satisfaction with, along with the overall outcome of, ED therapy. This study was significant because many past assessments were based on the *doctor's* perception of how well the medication worked. As may be expected, oral medication was the overall favorite; seventy-nine percent preferred to use an oral medication, even though only sixteen percent had satisfactory results. The oral medications used at the time were yohimbine and trazodone, which studies have since concluded are not effective.

The other treatments (tension bands, self-injection therapy, vacuum devices, and surgery) were each initially chosen by fewer than five percent of users. Satisfaction with the selected therapy in these small groups ranged from thirty-seven percent for the constrictive bands to one hundred percent for surgery (to implant a prosthesis). Eight percent elected not to have any therapy at all. Since the completion of this study, several effective oral and one intraurethral medication have been approved by the FDA and are available by prescription in the United States. Thus, the satisfaction curve reported may be shifted. In fact a currently practicing urologic surgeon estimates the satisfaction rate among patients receiving penile implants to be seventy to seventy-five percent.

After a two-year follow-up at the conclusion of the study, only forty percent of the patients were satisfied with their sexual function. Most of the sixty percent who were not satisfied "chose to avoid more effective therapies even if available." Although not highlighted at that time, the Jarow paper may have been the first to indicate what is now identified as the "drop-out rate."

The incredible demand for Viagra® confirmed the findings of this earlier study that oral medications are vastly preferred, even if other medications are available and more appropriate (e.g., would work better) for some men.

To have an erection using oral medications, a man must be sexually aroused. In fact, the effectiveness of these medications is somewhat proportional to the man's level of excitement. Vacuum devices, injections, or implants will produce an erection without the man being aroused.

Use of a medication may not have the expected results, either initially, after a few times, or at all. In other words, don't start doubting yourself if something does not work because no one miracle aid works for everybody. Try it a few times, see if there is an effect, ask your doctor to adjust the dosage, and, if it still doesn't work, ask the doctor to prescribe something else. Also ask your doctor if the prescribed product is a medication that becomes more effective over time. Men have commented anecdotally that this is the case with Viagra®. One study noted: "Early non-responders to sildenafil should not be disheartened, as they will more likely later respond."

Because applicability, suitability, and effectiveness vary for different people, some doctors prescribe "erection cocktails" (combinations of medications) for patients; some of these are discussed further later in this chapter and others are covered in Chapter 9. For example, one doctor prescribes an injection for one person, but an injected medication plus a pill for someone else. Patients trying combinations without medical consultation run the risk of serious side effects that may require emergency medical treatment. Only a doctor who knows your medical history should make this determination. You, your doctor, and your partner jointly should make any decision about what is best for you.

Understand the psychological side effects of treatment

With aids that are generally referred to as "performance medication," many men have newfound capability. Therefore, they must think about the consequences of using these products. If a medication does work, one consequence is that there may be more demands on one or both partners in the relationship. For example, in a relationship that has settled down to minimal or no sex for some time, how will the partners react to changing the balance? If the medication works, will one or both of the partners be happy and excited about the renewed capability—or afraid of the new sexual relationship?

Some partners may be afraid or at least not enthusiastic about returning to physical aspects of the early relationship if they have been living in a relationship where sex has been absent. We have been told about women asking their husband's doctor to stop prescribing erectile aids. The decision to use a certain medication and to continue using it should be made by both partners. Many ED specialists have commented that most of the time men come in for treatment without their partner. A partner who is unhappy with resuming sexual activity or using a specific medication may be responsible for the man's dissatisfaction and discontinuing therapy.

You need to realize that, when you had to face the fact that you had lost some or all of your erectile capability, you were affected psychologically. Now that you start thinking of being able to have erections again, you may feel good. On the other hand, you may feel uncertain and even anxious. You may even feel threatened because you are uncertain how your partner will react. Equally, your partner may feel threatened and start worrying about new demands being imposed.

Assuming you and your partner agree that you should use a commercial impotence therapy, realistic expectations should be the order of the day. The therapy may not work at all, may work some of the time, or may work partially, and many users report side effects. In other words, don't believe everything in the advertisements.

Understand what anxiety can do

Another possible effect is that anxiety may change the level of response and the time it takes for a medication to be effective. To say it again, anxiety influences the effectiveness of medication. Perhaps if both of you take a relaxed attitude ("Well, let's see what happens"), your anxiety will be minimized. Even if a medication is not entirely effective, as long as your anxiety is lessened, your natural ability can resurface more easily and may then be enhanced by the medication. In situations where men have erectile dysfunction, a percentage (generally thought to be about ten percent) improves with any medication, primarily because performance anxiety is relieved. Often, if a couple had a satisfactory physical relationship before prostate surgery or radiation, a "starting aid" is sufficient to get over the anxiety threshold. There is also the possibility of "anxiety override." A man concerned about whether he will have an erection and be able to perform may already know that his chronic anxiety will diminish any natural ability he has. Even when he takes a medication that could be effective, anxiety can completely suppress the effect of the medication.

The importance of a conservative approach

A conservative approach to therapy is usually advisable; some guidelines for a conservative approach are as follows:

• Begin with the least invasive therapy that both partners are willing to work with. Although a vacuum erection device is perhaps the least invasive therapy, if the couple feels that the spontaneity of their lovemaking would be disrupted by having to assemble and manipulate this large mechanical device, then this may not be the best choice as an initial treatment. As another example, if one partner is squeamish about needles, then injection therapy may be a poor starting choice for that couple.

• In the case of drugs, start with the lowest possible dosage. If the initial dose is not effective, gradually work up to a higher dose; however, only do this on the advice of your physician and do not exceed the maximum dose he or she recommends.

Any medication may have side effects. A new medication may have unexpected results. This is equivalent to deciding how much whiskey to give to a person who has never had liquor before. Some people would give them half a shot (the conservative approach), while others would give them a glassful. So try the minimum, and increase the dose as necessary. However, this requires a supportive partner who is willing to work with you and won't put you down if the low dosage does not work.

You need to work with your doctor regarding medication dosage. Guessing at the appropriate dosage may lead to problems. A doctor may make an exception to the rule of starting with the lowest strength when the patient or the couple has not benefited from other therapies. The doctor may prescribe a maximum dose to increase the probability of success. By having a successful sexual experience, the man's anxiety may be lessened in the future and erections may be obtained with a lower dose of medication.

The first use of injection medication should always occur in the doctor's office so that the medication can be adjusted, or "titrated." (Titration is the process of beginning with a certain amount of a chemical and adding known amounts until the point is reached at which the desired reaction occurs.) As an informed patient you should insist on this. A patient who opted to try injection therapy found out why this was so important. After receiving the injection, he developed an erection; however, the erection continued to swell and became quite painful; since he was in the doctor's office, treatment was immediately undertaken, sparing him a long painful episode and preventing damage to his penis. If the doctor is unwilling to do an initial injection during an office visit, find another doctor.

Always try to put the least burden on your system. Some medicines affect the way other medications work. Tell your doctor about *all* medicines, including all over-the-counter medication, herbal medication, or nutritional supplements you are taking before new drugs are prescribed. The prospective new medication may not be as effective or may conflict with other medications you are currently taking. The combination may worsen side effects of one or both of the medications, may be extremely harmful, or, in the worst case, could be fatal.

Why so much information?

We must say a word about our methodology for putting together the following information on specific treatments. We used a variety of sources, including product manufacturers and health care professionals, to gather our information. In some cases, information about a particular treatment was obtained from several sources. Most of the manufacturers commented on our write-up concerning their products. We allowed manufacturers to suggest changes that clarified a description or added new data from recently completed studies; we did not allow changing negative comments about products from either patients or doctors. As with any descriptions about fast moving medical trends, our information may not be entirely up-to-date at the time you read it; it is imperative that patients continue to do their own research and develop a relationship with a medical professional they can trust to bring them the best available information on the subject.

In addition, drug and device prices and other information were obtained from the manufacturers and from reputable Internet sites that were linked to the Web sites of a major pharmacy chain in the Washington, D.C. area. For various reasons, some information could not be obtained, and these instances have been noted as "not available." The prices noted are provided only as reference points. Prices will differ depending on the area of the country, the pharmacy, and other factors. Before you buy, it is okay, and even advisable, to ask your pharmacy about price and the portion covered by insurance.

Unfortunately, companies with New Drug Applications pending for Food and Drug Administration (FDA) approval are not permitted to release much information on these products. In these instances we have provided as much as we have been able to obtain. New products in development are noted here for information purposes only. There are probably others in the pipeline that we are not aware of.

We do not recommend or endorse any product. Since new information becomes available continually, information reported here might become outdated quickly. To minimize the chance of an adverse reaction, a physician must be included in the decision to pursue a medical therapy for erectile dysfunction. An individual's response to a medication is influenced by many factors, including genetics, overall health status, and other medications or supplements being taken. Therefore, you should not use the following information as the basis for any medical decision.

We provide much medical, medication/therapy, and product information because being an informed patient and consumer is essential to good health and optimal health care. However, the information is not presented for patients to treat themselves. Patients must consult with their doctors so that informed, joint decisions can be made. Doctors have the medical background and your history to work with in order to prescribe the best approach for your health care and quality of life.

You can help your doctor and yourself in discussing treatment options by requesting product prescribing information. This information is available in the form of package inserts. Some companies also provide a patient package insert written in nonscientific language. If you use the Internet, seek sites that will provide current and accurate information; manufacturers' Web sites are a good place to start (they sometimes post the package inserts for their drugs). Other good choices include the American Medical Association (*ama-assn.org*), Medscape (*medscape.com*), and the Web sites of major educational institutions and major hospitals.

Products listed here may be available in other countries though but not in the United States. The FDS says that drugs should not be purchased from sources outside the United States because of differing regulations regarding the safety and effectiveness of the drugs and because of differing laws governing manufacturing practices. Any medication should be purchased only with a prescription obtained after a *face-to-face* consultation with, and thorough physical examination by, a licensed physician. The doctor's exam may find a condition that the patient was not aware of, and that may alter the recommended treatment. Answering an online questionnaire to obtain a prescription from a "doctor" is neither an examination nor a consultation. Drugs should be purchased only from a properly licensed retailer or distributor in the United States.

During 2002 and 2003 the cost of medications skyrocketed. Purchasing medications from foreign countries or from Web sites purporting to sell "generic" or "equivalent" versions of approved drugs may be tempting but could place your health in jeopardy. These drugs may not contain the amount of medication indicated on their labels; they may have too much or too little, or they may not contain any active ingredient. They may contain fillers that are themselves potentially harmful. In addition they may be adulterated, intentionally or inadvertently, with compounds that may interact with your other medications or that may pose a direct health threat. These medications may not be labeled with an expiration date and they may have been subjected to improper storage conditions, such as extreme heat or cold. Always be wary of deeply discounted drug prices from an Internet site or from TV or magazine ads; chances are good that you will not get what you think you are paying for.

Pill Splitting

Another point that merits discussion is pill splitting, because it is discussed on ED email lists. If several different strengths of a medication are available and they all cost about the same amount per pill, it may seem logical to purchase, for example, fifty-milligram tablets of a medication and split them in half so that you have twenty-five-milligram doses. Some health plans are even advocating this practice. This is not a good idea, however, since the active ingredient (chemical) may not be evenly distributed throughout the pill, so even if you are very precise when you split the tablet, you may not receive two equal doses. It is very difficult to be precise when splitting tablets, even if you use a pill-splitter designed for that very use. This may be one reason that men find one half-strength pill does not work as well as another half-strength pill.

Also, some pills have a coating that may be a factor in where and how the medication is absorbed in the stomach and intestinal tract. Splitting the pill breaks the coating and may alter the place and rate of the drug's absorption, which in turn may alter the effectiveness or produce side effects.

Thus, we reiterate: It is *your* responsibility to consult with a licensed health care provider before undertaking any type of treatment for erectile dysfunction. Any medication should be obtained using a prescription obtained only after an in-person consultation with a physician and purchased from a reputable U.S. retailer.

Interpreting Clinical Trial Results

A brief definition of clinical trial phases is included here to help clarify the process of developing new drugs. It is important to note that early trials use young, healthy men who take a single dose of the drug being studied. Specific parameters are then measured to understand such aspects as how well the drug is absorbed when given by different methods (orally or by injection for example), how long the drug remains in the body, how it is removed from the body, and so on. During the later phases, the findings may indicate that the drug does not work each time, that it may require more time to become effective, or that it may lose effectiveness with repeated use.

Phase I—Studies that involve a small group of people who all take the same drug but by different routes of administration and/or different dosages. This phase tests the safety and dosage of the drug.

Phase II (or 2)—These studies focus on comparing the new treatment with the current standard treatment or placebo. Larger than phase I studies, phase II studies continue to test the drug for safety and efficacy.

Phase III (or 3)—These are large trials that randomize patients to test the effects of the new treatment without bias from researchers. Phase III studies test the effectiveness of the drug as well as potential side effects. Safety of the drug also is monitored.

Phase IV (or 4)—These studies occur after the FDA has approved the drug for use in the United States. Phase IV studies usually concentrate on possible new indications or long-term effect of the drug. These studies may include testing use in specific groups such as children or the elderly.

In this chapter and in Chapter 9, we frequently quote statistics from the clinical trials presented by the pharmaceutical companies. But what does it really mean when a drug is reported to have a success rate of, for example, seventy-five percent? Or that fifty percent of men reported improvement?

The key is in the definition of the terms "success" or "improvement" within the context of the particular clinical trial. In general, clinical trials are designed with specific inclusion and exclusion criteria for the patients, and well-defined endpoints for therapeutic outcome, or response. As an example of patient selection criteria, Dr. John P. Mulhall, Director, Sexual Medicine Programs, Cornell-New York Medical Center, in an article in the August 2003 issue of the *Journal of Urology*, states, "85% of all patients enrolled in phase III trials … have been white." Thus the data may not be applicable to African-American, Hispanic, or Asian men. Additionally, "There has been a trend to exclude from oral erectogenic agent trials patients who have undergone radical prostatectomy or pelvic radiation therapy, as many of these patients, depending on the interval since treatment, are poorer responders to oral agents and may compromise efficacy data."

One end point frequently used is the answer to certain questions on the International Index of Erectile Function (IIEF), a questionnaire that is highly validated for use in these clinical trials. This is a self-administered questionnaire, and in some cases does not accurately distinguish between organic and psychogenic ED. Since efficacy of investigational drugs is measured based highly on the organic nature of ED, this failure could lead to misinterpretation of the efficacy data. Each answer on the questionnaire is assigned a point value with lower scores indicating more severe ED, and an improvement of a defined number of points is considered clinically meaningful. Therefore, an improvement from a designation of severe to a designation of moderate would be considered meaningful; however, this does not necessarily mean that that patient can achieve or maintain an erection rigid enough for intercourse.

Thus, approval of new ED drugs may be based on the clinically meaningful improvement reported by the researcher, while the patient may interpret the numbers to mean achievement of a rigid erection suitable for intercourse. So bear in mind that the success rate reported in clinical trials may not match your definition of success.

The List of Treatments

The discussion in this chapter of the means for improving the ability to obtain and maintain erections includes all medications in one group and all devices, including prostheses or implants, treated separately. Penile rehabilitation as a therapy can be achieved by several different means and is therefore discussed separately from the others. Within the next five to seven years, some new research routes may yield equally or more effective means for obtaining erections. An overview of some of these new research directions is included. Here is a list of the treatments discussed:

• Penile rehabilitation
• Oral medications

- Intraurethral medication
- Penile injection (intracavernosal injection)
- Topical medications: penile creams and gels
- New products in development
- Devices
  - Penile splints and supports
  - Vacuum erection devices
  - Penile implants
- Surgery and neural therapies
  - Nerve sparing surgery
  - Nerve grafting surgery
  - Penile vascular surgery
- New target areas for erectile dysfunction research

Table 8.1 lists the medications discussed in this section. Table 8.2 lists the devices.

Penile rehabilitation

Patients who have had pelvic surgery within six months of reading this book may be especially interested in this section. Physicians implement this therapy using different options to counter possible impotence effects of surgery and thereby possibly improve erections. There is no clear indication whether penile rehabilitation will aid patients who are more than six months postoperative.

Until relatively recently, urologists counseled their prostatectomy patients to wait six months to a year after surgery to see if erectile function would return. After that interval, the doctor would then prescribe injections (in the pre-Viagra® days) or, since 1998, either Viagra® or injections. A study in 1995 indicated that using vacuum therapy improved nocturnal erections, which are considered essential to maintaining overall penile health. In 1997, Dr. Francesco Montorsi and his colleagues explored the idea that giving intracavernosal injections of alprostadil soon after surgery would improve the chances for recovering potency following radical prostatectomy. The production of erections at regular intervals and not for the purpose of intercourse, using vacuum or drug therapy, is referred to as *penile rehabilitation*. The aim of this

Table 8-1. Medications Listed in Alphabetical Order by Manufacturer

Brand Name	Generic Name	Route of Administration	Manufacturer	Page No.
Levitra®	vardenafil	Oral	Bayer	115
Cialis®	tadalafil	Oral	ICOS	117
Topiglan®[1]	alprostadil	Topical	MacroChem	128
Alprox-TD®	alprostadil	Topical	NexMed	129
Viagra®	sildenafil	Oral	Pfizer	120
Caverject®	alprostadil	Intracavernosal injection	Pfizer	139
EDEX®	alprostadil	Intracavernosal injection	Schwarz Pharma	140
Invicorp™[2]	alprostadil	Intracavernosal injection	Senetek	142
Uprima[2]	apomorphine	Sublingual (under the tongue)	TAP	125
yohimbine	yohimbine	Oral	various	123
MUSE®	alprostadil	Intraurethral insertion	Vivus	132
Vasomax[1]	phentolamine	Oral	Zonagen	126

[1]New drug under investigation; not yet available
[2]Not available in the United States

therapy is to increase the amount of oxygenated blood brought into the cavernous tissue of the penis, thus providing nourishment to the erectile tissue and promoting penile health.

A study, sponsored by Pfizer, and reported in April 2003, indicated that in a group of men given sildenafil (Viagra®) nightly for nine months, beginning four weeks after nerve sparing prostatectomy, twenty-seven percent (fourteen out of a group of fifty-one) showed an increase of spontaneous erections compared with four percent (one out of twenty-five) in a control group of patients who did not receive sildenafil therapy. It must be noted that men taking nitrate medication would not be able to utilize oral therapy with any PDE-5 inhibitor, such as sildenafil (Viagra®), vardenafil (Levitra®), or tadalafil (Cialis®) due to the possibility of dangerous drug interactions between these types of medication.

Table 8-2. Devices Listed in Alphabetical Order by Manufacturer

Brand Name	Type	Description	Manufacturer	Page No.
AMS 700CX/CXR	Prosthesis	3-part inflatable	American Medical Systems	160
AMS 700 Ultrex/Ultrex Plus	Prosthesis	3-part inflatable	American Medical Systems	160
AMS Ambicor	Prosthesis	2-part inflatable	American Medical Systems	160
AMS Malleable 600M/650M	Prosthesis	Malleable	American Medical Systems	160
Rejoyn Support Sleeve	Penile support	Latex external support	American MedTech	147
Touch® II	Vacuum erection device	Battery; use with Sure Release Tension System	Augusta Medical Systems	151
Response® II	Vacuum erection device	Manual; use with Sure Release Tension System	Augusta Medical Systems	151
ErecAid™ Esteem™	Vacuum erection device	Battery and manual models available; use with Pressure Point Tension Rings	Endocare	156
Alpha® I	Prosthesis	3-part inflatable	Mentor	161
Titan™	Prosthesis	3-part inflatable	Mentor	161
Acu-Form®	Prosthesis	Malleable	Mentor	161
Rejoyn Vacuum Therapy System	Vacuum erection device	Manual; use with support rings	Pos-T-Vac	155
MVP–700 System	Vacuum erection device	Manual; use with thermoplastic elastomer tension rings	Pos-T-Vac	155
IVP–600 Vacuum Therapy System	Vacuum erection device	Manual; use with tension rings	Pos-T-Vac	155
Actis®	Constriction band	Adjustable constriction band	Vivus	133, 140

Intracavernosal injections (injections into the erection chambers of the penis, called the corpora cavernosa) of alprostadil, and intraurethral administration of alprostadil have also been used for rehabilitation.

Vacuum therapy is another option, and at least one company provides a protocol for using their device as part of a penile rehabilitation regimen. Since vacuum therapy is a noninvasive, local therapy, it is safe for men taking medications that would preclude them from using a drug for rehabilitation therapy.

Bear in mind several points when considering a penile rehabilitation program. Generally, it has been suggested to begin rehabilitation four to six weeks after surgery, but be sure to have your doctor's approval before you begin any program; you don't want to disrupt the healing of the surgical site. There are no studies indicating if rehabilitation is of any benefit if it is begun six months or longer after surgery. If planning to use one of the drug therapies, be sure you do not take a higher dose than prescribed, and do not take any medication more frequently than prescribed. All the medications currently available state that there must be at least twenty-four hours between doses; some of the drugs are also limited to three uses per week. And if you are taking any other medications, you may not be a candidate for a drug-based rehabilitation program.

Use of a vacuum device is not limited to once in twenty-four hours, and one therapy protocol recommends using vacuum therapy twice daily for rehabilitation. Cost is also a consideration. Although the initial outlay for a vacuum therapy system may be as much as five hundred dollars, there are no additional costs associated with this type of therapy. Costs for drug-based therapy may appear to be less, but they are ongoing. At approximately ten dollars per pill and one pill per day, treatment for one month would be three hundred dollars. (Remember, in the study using sildenafil [Viagra®] reported here patients used the drug every night for nine months.)

If you have been recently diagnosed with prostate or other pelvic cancer, or if you have been recently treated, penile rehabilitation is an option worth considering. Although reported studies are still few, there is early support for its effectiveness and, at this time, no reported ill effects.

Oral medications

In mid-1998, many men found a new deity, the goddess Viagra®. The impact of this pill was rather well expressed in a urologist's Christmas letter we received: "John's year has been dominated by that little blue pill, Viagra®."

Viagra®, approved in mid-1998, was the first pill for erectile dysfunction to reach the market. Another pill, Levitra®, became available in August 2003. A third new oral drug, Cialis®, received FDA approval in November 2003. These drugs have become the first-line therapy of choice for treating ED; all work by inhibiting PDE-5, an enzyme that causes the erection to go down. Here are some important points to keep in mind when considering an oral medication to treat ED:

- "These drugs do not increase desire. All they do is help a man who already has the desire for sex to achieve an erection." This comment is issued by Pfizer for Viagra®, but it applies to all currently known oral medications. If you become "turned off," you will lose the erection.

- Oral erection medications should not be used more than once a day, and there should be at least twenty-four hours between doses, if the patient plans to use the drug on consecutive days.

- These drugs produce erections, not orgasms. Also, none of these drugs facilitate repeated orgasms. As we get older, the period between orgasms (refractory period) increases, and the ability to have orgasms decreases. However, Viagra® is reported to make it easier to have an orgasm.

- The high cost of oral medication and the fact that the price is the same regardless of strength may prompt some men to split the pill. Men who buy a higher strength and then split the pill should read the section on pill splitting in the introduction to this chapter.

Another prescription oral product, yohimbine, has debatable efficacy. The following pages present currently available information on these oral medications. The products are presented in alphabetical order by manufacturer in two parts. First are the products currently available in the United States, followed by those under development or available outside the United States.

Yohimbine is listed under its generic name (following Viagra®) because there are many manufacturers.

AVAILABLE IN THE UNITED STATES:

- Levitra® (vardenafil)   Bayer
- Cialis® (tadalafil)   Lilly-ICOS
- Viagra® (sildenafil)   Pfizer
- yohimbine (various names)   various manufacturers

AVAILABLE OUTSIDE THE UNITED STATES OR UNDER DEVELOPMENT

- Uprima® (apomorphine)   Tap Pharmaceutical Products, Inc.
- Vasomax (phentolamine)   Zonagen

Note: Viagra®, Levitra®, and Cialis® are all classified as PDE-5 inhibitors. Phosphodiesterase type 5 (PDE-5) is an enzyme that plays a major role in maintaining erections. In men with erectile dysfunction it has been found that inhibiting this enzyme allows the erection to occur and be maintained. Because these drugs have many similarities in their chemical structure, there are also similarities in the side effects and drug interactions of these drugs. The main caution to be aware of is that *no one* taking nitrate medication should take these drugs. This is true even if you take the medication only occasionally ("as needed"). The interaction of these two types of medication can cause a sudden drop in blood pressure, and the results may be fatal.

Although these drugs primarily inhibit PDE-5, they do have some effect on other PDEs that occur in many other body tissues. Of particular concern is PDE-6, which occurs in the retina of the eye. Men with retinitis pigmentosa or other eye diseases involving the retina are at greater risk of damage to the eyes if they take these drugs. Men with retinal disease were excluded from trials of these drugs because of the risk of permanent eye damage. Inform your doctor of any eye problems you have before deciding to use an oral PDE-5 inhibitor to treat ED.

Manufacturer: Bayer

Brand Name: Levitra®

Active Chemical: vardenafil HCl

Dosage: 2.5-, 5-, 10-, 20-mg tablets

Administration: The recommended starting dose is 10 mg. This may be increased to a maximum recommended dose of 20 mg or decreased to 5 mg, based on efficacy and side effects. The maximum recommended dosing frequency is once per day and doses should be at least 24 hours apart. This drug may be taken with or without food, and should be taken approximately 60 minutes before sexual activity. Although not specifically addressed in the prescribing information for Levitra®, drinking alcohol can increase the chance of headache, dizziness, increased heart rate, or lower blood pressure, and therefore alcohol should be used with care when taking this drug. Sexual stimulation is necessary for a response to treatment.

Status: Available in the United States since August 2003; available in Europe since March 2003

Price: Pharmacy price in the Washington, D.C. area is approximately $12.00 per pill for 10 mg, $13.00 for 20 mg

Warnings: Levitra® must not be used if you are taking nitrate medications, either regularly or on an as-needed basis. Nitrate medications are frequently used to treat angina, a symptom of heart disease which can cause pain in the chest, jaw, or down the arm. These medications include nitroglycerin in any dose form (tablets, sprays, ointments, pastes, or patches), as well as some recreational drugs often called "poppers" (amyl nitrate, butyl nitrate). Any medication with any form of the word "nitrate" in its generic name (such as mononitrate, dinitrate) is a nitrate medication; Levitra® should not be taken with any of these medications. Check with your doctor or pharmacist if you are not sure whether any of your medications contain nitrates.

Do not take Levitra® if you take any medication called an "alpha-blocker"; such medication is used to treat high blood pressure or prostate problems. Examples of alpha-blockers include Hytrin (terazosin), Flomax (tamsulosin), Cardura (doxazosin), Minipress (prazosin), and Uroxatral (alfuzosin). This is not a complete list, so be sure to tell your doctor *all* the medications you are taking if you are considering a prescription for Levitra®.

An additional safety concern that is sometimes overlooked by this patient population is their ability to safely engage in sexual activity with or without Levitra® therapy. Many men in our generation, especially those with multiple underlying health problems, may not have been engaging in any regular physical activity (and probably not in sex). Now, with the potential for them to again engage in sexual relations because of Levitra® therapy, they should be evaluated by their doctor to determine their ability to tolerate the physical exertion that is part of any sexual activity.

Side Effects: During clinical trials the most commonly reported side effects for Levitra® were headache (15 percent), facial flushing (11 percent), runny nose (9 percent), and indigestion (4 percent). Occurrence of these side effects generally decreased over time. Rare side effects include seeing a blue tinge to objects or difficulty distinguishing between the colors blue and green.

Comments: If you have been advised not to engage in sexual activity due to any type of health problem, you should not take Levitra®. Sexual activity may place a strain on your heart, especially if you have any type of heart disease or have had a heart attack.

Levitra®, at a dose of 20 mg, was effective in 79 percent of patients with mild ED and in 39 percent of patients with severe ED. In one study (sponsored by Bayer and GlaxoSmithKline), nearly half (46.1 percent) of men with unsatisfactory results using Viagra®, were successful when given Levitra®.

As is true for all the PDE-5 inhibitors, Levitra® is not an aphrodisiac. It will not cause an erection to occur unless the man is sexually aroused.

For more information: 800-468-0894

Web site: *www.levitra.com*

Manufacturer: Lilly-ICOS
Brand Name: Cialis®
Active Chemical: tadalafil
Dosage: 5- and 20-mg tablets

Administration: The recommended starting dose for most men is 10 mg. Cialis® may be taken with or without meals. Alcohol should not be drunk in excess when taking Cialis®; alcohol can increase your chances of headache, dizziness, increased heart rate, or lower blood pressure. Cialis® may become effective as soon as 30 minutes after it is taken, and may improve the ability to have sexual activity for up to 36 hours. Sexual stimulation is necessary for a response to treatment.

Status: Received FDA approval for marketing in the United States in November 2003 and became available in January 2004. Available in more than forty countries including countries in Europe, Australia, New Zealand, Brazil, Mexico, Russia, Singapore, and Saudi Arabia.

Price: Approximate price range is $9.00–$11.00 per tablet, regardless of size.

Warnings: Cialis® must not be used if you are taking nitrate medications, either regularly or on an as-needed basis. Nitrate medications are frequently used to treat angina, a symptom of heart disease which can cause pain in the chest, jaw, or down the arm. These medications include nitroglycerin in any dose form (tablets, sprays, ointments, pastes, or patches), as well as some recreational drugs often called "poppers" (amyl nitrate, butyl nitrate). Any medication with any form of the word "nitrate" in its generic name (such as mononitrate, dinitrate) is a nitrate medication; Cialis® should not be taken with any of these medications. Check with your doctor or pharmacist if you are not sure whether any of your medications contain nitrates.

Do not use Cialis® if you take any medication called an "alpha blocker," *except* Flomax at a dose of 0.4 mg daily. These medications are used for treating prostate problems and high blood pressure and include Hytrin (terazosin), Flomax (tamsulosin), Cardura (doxazosin), Minipress (prazosin), and Uroxatral (alfuzosin). This is not a complete list, so be sure to tell your doctor *all* the medications you are taking if you are considering a prescription for Cialis®. Flomax at a dose of 0.4 mg per day is safe to take when using Cialis®; however, other alpha-blockers may cause a sudden drop in blood pressure, resulting in dizziness or fainting.

An additional safety concern that is sometimes overlooked by this patient population is their ability to safely engage in sexual activity with or without Cialis® therapy. Many men in our generation, especially those with multiple underlying disease problems, may not have been engaging in any regular physical activity (and probably not in sex). Now, with the potential for them to again engage in sexual relations because of Cialis® therapy, they should be evaluated by their doctor to determine their ability to tolerate the physical exertion that is part of any sexual activity.

Side Effects: The most commonly reported side effects are headache, flushing, upset stomach, muscle pain, and backache. Some are higher with Cialis® than Viagra® (e.g. headache [11.2 percent vs. 8.8 percent for Viagra®], which could be mild to moderate in intensity, upset stomach [6 percent percent for Cialis® vs. 4.2 percent for Viagra®], and common coldlike symptoms [4.7 percent for Cialis® and 2.8 percent for Viagra®].) Muscle ache and nasal congestion were worse for Viagra® than Cialis®.

Comments: If you have been advised not to engage in sexual activity due to any type of health problem, you should not take Cialis®. Sexual activity may place a strain on your heart, especially if you have any type of heart disease or have had a heart attack.

One study of men who had undergone bilateral nerve sparing prostatectomy showed that 62 percent had improved erections and more than half of all participants had successful intercourse. Several studies showed that up to 79 percent of men had improved erections with Cialis®. Another study showed that 67 percent of men reported being able to have successful intercourse after taking Cialis® for the first time. Other studies have shown that Cialis® may be effective for up to 36 hours. However, studies only involved a single attempt at intercourse during this time period.

There are few studies comparing Cialis® with other PDE-5 inhibitors. One study published in November 2003 (prior to FDA approval for Cialis®) sought "to determine what proportion of ED patients currently taking Viagra® would, after a period of treatment with Cialis®, elect to resume treatment with Viagra® or elect to switch to Cialis® 20 mg. for a longer period."

The 47 men participating in the study were already undergoing ED treatment with Viagra® at fixed doses of 25, 50, or 100 mg, for at least six weeks and up to 24 weeks. They were then given 20 mg of Cialis®. for nine weeks. All of the men were given three weeks of Viagra® after enrolling in the study. After a "washout period" they were given the Cialis®.

They were then given the opportunity to choose their preferred treatment for a six-month extension during which they would receive their ED treatment free of charge. The result: 90.5 percent of the men who had previously used Viagra® preferred to continue treatment with Cialis®. The remaining 9.5 percent of the men opted for Viagra®.

In another study to determine patient preference for Cialis® 20 mg or Viagra® 50 mg, 66 percent of the men preferred Cialis® over Viagra®.

As is true for all the PDE-5 inhibitors, Cialis® is not an aphrodisiac. It will not cause an erection to occur unless the man is sexually aroused.

For more information: 877-CIALIS-1 (877-242-5471)

Web site: *www.cialis.com*

Manufacturer: Pfizer

Brand Name: Viagra®

Active Chemical: Sildenafil citrate

Dosage: 25-, 50-, 100-mg tablets

Administration: The maximum dose that can be taken in one day is 100 mg. The pill must be taken on an empty stomach (at least two hours after a meal), and after taking the pill you should wait about one hour before lovemaking. A low-fat meal is best. Food and fat delay and reduce intestinal absorption, thereby reducing the drug's effectiveness. The man should not use alcohol when taking Viagra®. The drug will take effect within 30–60 minutes in most patients. The increased ability to have an erection may last up to four hours. Sexual stimulation is necessary for a response to treatment.

Status: Available since April 1998

Price: $8–$9 per pill regardless of dosage

Warnings: Viagra® must *not* be used if you are taking nitrate medications, either regularly or on an as-needed basis. Nitrate medications are frequently used to treat angina, a symptom of heart disease which can cause pain in the chest, jaw, or down the arm. These medications include nitroglycerin in any dose form (tablets, sprays, ointments, pastes, or patches), as well as some recreational drugs often called "poppers" (amyl nitrate, butyl nitrate). Any medication with any form of the word nitrate in its generic name (such as mononitrate, dinitrate) is a nitrate medication; Viagra® should not be taken with any of these medications. Check with your doctor or pharmacist if you are not sure whether any of your medications contain nitrates. Most of the 138 fatalities associated with taking the drug in 1998 were in patients taking Viagra® who disregarded the warnings about the drug's conflict with nitrate medication. Therefore, if you take any nitrate medication, even if prescribed only on an "as needed" basis, you should not be using Viagra®.

Viagra®, in doses greater than 25 mg, should not be taken within 4 hours of taking an alpha-blocker (used for treating high blood pressure and prostate problems); examples are Cardura (doxazosin), Minipress (prazosin), Hytrin (terazosin), and Flomax (tamsulosin).

An additional safety concern that is sometimes overlooked by this patient population is their ability to safely engage in sexual activity with or without Viagra® therapy. Many men in our generation, especially those with multiple underlying health problems, may not have been engaging in any regular physical activity (and probably not in sex). Now, with the potential for them to again engage in sexual relations because of Viagra® therapy, they should be evaluated by their doctor to determine their ability to tolerate the physical exertion that is part of any sexual activity. As the Pfizer patient summary puts it, "Ask your doctor if your heart is healthy enough to handle the extra strain of having sex. If you have chest pains, dizziness, or nausea during sex, stop having sex and immediately call your doctor."

Side Effects: The most common side effects include headache (16 percent) (similar to coital headaches), facial flushing (10 percent), stomach upset or nausea (7 percent), and some sinus difficulty including nasal congestion (4 percent).

The most publicized side effect is a blue-green haze and increased perception of bright light several hours after taking Viagra® that affected 3 percent of patients in the clinical trials. This effect was reported more frequently at the higher dose of 100 mg.

Comments: If you have been advised not to engage in sexual activity due to any type of health problem, you should not take Viagra®. Sexual activity may place a strain on your heart, especially if you have any type of heart disease or have had a heart attack.

However, an analysis of 130 clinical trials involving more than 12,000 men showed no difference in the incidence of heart attacks or other heart-related deaths between patients who received Viagra® and those who were given a placebo. If you are able to engage in physical activities comparably strenuous to intercourse, and have no other contraindications (such as use of nitrate medication; see "Warnings"); Viagra® may be an option.

Men should begin with a low dosage, and try it three times (not in one day nor on three consecutive days) before discussing increasing the dosage with their doctor. Viagra® improves erections and is reported to enhance orgasm.

In four studies lasting 12 to 24 weeks each and involving 1,797 patients, improvement was reported by 63 percent of men taking 25 mg, 74 percent taking 50 mg, and 82 percent of those taking 100 mg; 24 percent of patients receiving placebo reported improvement. Patients in these studies all had documented erectile dysfunction from a variety of causes, excluding only spinal cord injury.

Across all trials, 43 percent of radical prostatectomy patients had improved erections using Viagra®, compared with 15 percent given placebo.

Response to Viagra® is affected by the presence or absence of the neurovascular bundles (i.e., nerve sparing versus non-nerve sparing surgical procedure). Patients who had undergone bilateral nerve sparing surgery had a response rate of 71.7 percent, those who had been treated with a unilateral nerve sparing procedure showed a 50 percent positive response, and those with non-nerve sparing surgery had a 15.4 percent response.

Effectiveness is supposedly better for radiation patients. In a study of patients treated by external beam radiation therapy, Viagra® was effective in about 50 percent of the men. Most of the patients required the higher dose of 100 mg. Other studies have reported effectiveness rates up to 71 percent in radiation patients. Patients taking Lupron can have erections with Viagra® and so can orchiectomy patients.

Although it has been suggested that tolerance (the patient finds that the dose must be increased in order to achieve the same effect) to sildenafil may occur, this has not been scientifically established. Carefully following the administration guidelines with regard to both the dose and the timing (at least two hours after a meal) will maximize the success of the treatment.

Viagra® may also be prescribed in combination with a vacuum therapy device and/or tension rings, such as Actis®. Before using any combination of therapies, consult your doctor.

As previously mentioned, no erection will occur unless you are aroused. Taking the pill and reading the newspaper until there is an erection means that you are in for a long reading session. It will not happen. Similarly, if you are aroused and have an erection, but are suddenly distracted or think about how your stocks went down that day, so will the erection. However, since the effects of the drug that allow the man the capability to get an erection may last for up to four hours, if there is a low moment, the couple can try later on. The maximum recommended dosing frequency is once per day.

For more information: 888-4VIAGRA (888-484-2472)

Web site: *www.viagra.com*

Active Chemical: Yohimbine

Manufacturer: Many, such as Duramed, Palisades Pharmaceutical, and others

Brand Names: Actibine, Aphrodyne, Baron-X, Dayto Himbin, PMS-Yohimbine, Prohim, Thybine, Yocon, Yohlmar, Yohimex, Yoman, Yovital

Dosage: Each tablet contains 5.4 mg yohimbine

Administration: 1 tablet 2–4 times daily

Status: Available with prescription only. (Yohimbine is a controlled substance.)

Price: Varies

Side Effects: Anxiety, increase in blood pressure, nervousness, dizziness

Comments: Yohimbine, obtained from the bark of a tree, is marketed in a number of products for bodybuilding and "enhanced male performance" and has been rumored to be an aphrodisiac for many years. The chemical seems more effective in patients with psychologically based impotence than in those with an organic basis. Yohimbine has enjoyed a reputation in spite of studies that have shown that yohimbine was "not significantly better than placebo in restoring potency" based on a statistical analysis. One study showed that 21 percent of patients taking yohimbine medication recovered their sexual function compared with 13.8 percent of the patients taking a placebo. When researchers increased the dose in another study, they found that 14 percent of the men became potent again (Spark, p. 283). Despite poor results, yohimbine is often prescribed because it has relatively mild side effects. If yohimbine "works," it begins to do so two to three weeks after the patient begins to take it.

Since the same percentage in both groups of patients, the control group and the treated groups, showed results, it appears that the men seemed to respond to the information provided by clinicians that were testing the drug's ability to help men recover their erectile function (a classic placebo effect).

Because the "response" to the drug is relatively quick, "many physicians now feel comfortable offering men with psychogenic impotence a one month trial of yohimbine to determine whether they will, or will not notice a return of satisfactory penile erections."

A sufficient number of studies have been done and their results conflict. One study concluded that the benefits of using yohimbine outweigh the risks and suggested that it "remain a viable option for men with erectile dysfunction" (*Journal of Urology*, July 1998). Another small study found that 50 percent of participants "were successful in completing intercourse in more than 75 percent of attempts." The men in this study who responded positively had less severe erectile dysfunction as determined by several measures. The authors concluded that "yohimbine is an effective therapy to treat organic erectile dysfunction in some men with erectile dysfunction" (Abstract, *International Journal of Impotence Research*, 2002).

It is widely reported that yohimbine causes minimal side effects, and these are somewhat the same as with other oral medications: anxiety, increased heart rate and blood pressure, dizziness, flushing, nausea, and headache. These side effects are said to be transient and will wear off after the drug is dissipated. A 1998 analysis of seven clinical trials showed that side effects were infrequent and reversible. Yohimbine should not be used by patients that have cardiac, hepatic, or renal disease. The active chemical causes vasodilation, which lowers blood pressure. At high doses, yohimbine should be avoided by individuals with hypotension (low blood pressure), diabetes, and heart, liver, or kidney disease. Yohimbine can cause serious adverse effects when taken with certain kinds of foods such as liver, cheeses, and red wine, over-the-counter nasal decongestants, and diet aids. Users must strictly avoid these types of foods and products. Symptoms of overdosage include weakness and nervous stimulation followed by paralysis, fatigue, stomach disorders, and ultimately death.

Although yohimbine sales are high, that does not mean it works. Ineffective substances often have the greatest sales when there is a perception that they have minimal side effects.

For more information: Search for yohimbine on the Internet.

Manufacturer: Abbott International and Takeda Chemical Industries, LTD (Japan)

Brand Names: Uprima® and Ixense

Active Chemical: Apomorphine

Dosage: 2 and 3 mg, not available in the United States

Administration: The pill is to be taken sublingually (dissolved under the tongue).

Status: *Not available in United States;* TAP, an Abbott and Takeda joint venture failed to win FDA approval in late summer 2003 and will not seek U.S. approval again. Available in Europe, Latin America (Uprima®), and Asia (Ixense) since 2001.

Price: Not available

Side Effects: The major side effects reported are nausea, headache, and dizziness.

Comments: Uprima®, a dopamine agonist, is designed to work in the central nervous system, using the body's natural pathways to produce an erection. It stimulates the brain center for sexual response, which then transmits the message down the spinal cord to produce an erection. The drug is designed to work on men with mild to moderate erectile dysfunction.

Data from three Phase III clinical trials reported at the 1999 American Urological Association (AUA) meeting showed that Uprima® "can increase the number of successful intercourse attempts." The studies used four dosage levels. The level of successful intercourse increased from 44 percent of the men at the lowest dosage, 2 mg, to 61 percent at 4 mg. The company also reported that the most common side effect was mild to moderate nausea.

For more information: 800-348-2779

Web site: *www.tap.com*

Manufacturer: Zonagen

Brand Name: Vasomax

Active Chemical: Phentolamine, an alpha-blocker, opens the blood vessels in the vascular smooth muscles of the penis to help restore normal function in approximately 15 minutes with normal sexual stimulation.

Dosage: Information not available

Administration: Information not available

Status: Applied for FDA approval

Price: Not available

Side Effects: Not available

Comments: In 1999, the company filed a New Drug Application for FDA approval and was therefore precluded from providing any current information. Previously available information showed that in a 148-patient Phase II clinical trial in Mexico, the drug worked on 42 percent of the men in every attempt. Two U.S. Phase III trials showed improvement in 34 percent and 40 percent of the men. There were some circulatory side effects. Zonagen then conducted additional, large open label studies with Vasomax.

Phentolamine has been around for a long time, and its effectiveness has been disputed. Its effectiveness is apparently due to its being a combined alpha-1 and alpha-2 blocker. Its current formulation permits the body to absorb it, whereas the body did not retain other formulations.

Zonagen's license for worldwide marketing rights to Schering Plough (signed in November 1997) was terminated by mutual agreement in July 2002.

In August 1999, the Food and Drug Administration (FDA) placed further clinical trials of Zonagen's phentolamine-based drugs (including Vasomax) on hold until "issues surrounding the Company's two-year rat study are satisfactorily resolved. FDA allowed Zonagen to complete the ... ongoing 12-week study in humans of Vasomax for erectile dysfunction." Three years later, in November 2002, the FDA notified Zonagen that an additional two-year animal study is required to lift the clinical hold on Vasomax.

For more information: The company does not wish to be contacted while drug is under FDA review.

Web site: *www.zonagen.com*

Topical medications: penile creams and gels

Topical medications include gels and creams that are applied directly to the head, or the glans, of the penis. We are aware of two topical products under development: Vaseline-type or creamlike products. The competitive advantage offered by topical medications is that they "could offer doctors a safer alternative to oral : pills," which have a whole-body (systemic) effect. Because they are easy to use, this class of products may be a more acceptable alternative to injections and MUSE®. In the course of developing these products, due diligence demands that companies also investigate possible effects on partners since these medications are applied to the skin. None of the products are currently available in the United States.

The following products are presented in alphabetical order by manufacturer.

• Topiglan® (alprostadil)   Macrochem
• Alprox-TD® (alprostadil)   NexMed

Manufacturer: MacroChem

Brand Name: Topiglan®

Active Chemical: Alprostadil

Dosage: Information not available

Administration: This is an investigational topical cream of alprostadil (the active ingredient in currently marketed Caverject®, EDEX, and MUSE®), combined with a proprietary skin penetration enhancer, SEPA®. After Topiglan® is applied to the penis using the fingertip shortly before intercourse, SEPA transiently fluidizes the lipids (fats) in penile skin to allow alprostadil absorption into local blood vessels to cause an erection.

Status: In Phase II clinical trials

Price: Not available

Side Effects: Information not available

Comments: Topiglan® cream is applied to the penis and appears to act locally. By comparison, medications taken orally circulate throughout the body and have the potential to cause side effects in other tissues and organs. In clinical trials completed to date, neither Topiglan®-treated patients nor their partners have displayed any remarkable systemic side effects. A 550-patient Phase II/III in-home clinical trial of Topiglan® gel was recently completed. While the subpopulation of protocol-conforming patients showed a statistically significant improvement in their erectile function and their ability to complete intercourse, the larger intent-to-treat population (which included patients who dropped out of the study) missed statistical significance in primary efficacy endpoints. Local intolerance of the gel reported by some men prompted a reformulation effort by MacroChem, and a new Topiglan® cream has demonstrated improved tolerance in a Phase I clinical trial. A Phase II office efficacy study was initiated in June 2003.

For more information: 781-862-4003

Web site: *www.macrochem.com*

Manufacturer: NexMed, Inc.

Brand Name: Alprox-TD®

Active Chemical: Alprostadil (prostaglandin E-1)

Dosage: Phase III clinical studies indicate safety and efficacy at dosages of 200 and 300 μg (micrograms). The commercial dose has not been selected.

Administration: A very small amount (approximately 100 mg) of cream is applied directly onto the tip of the penis at least 5–30 minutes before intercourse from a novel, easy-to-use single-dose applicator. Rapid absorption is obtained using the patented NexACT skin penetration enhancement technology

Status: In clinical trials. The results of Phase III studies are in press. Alprostadil topical cream is available in Asia under the tradename Befar; however, this is not exactly the same formulation as Alprox-TD®, which will be the product sold in the United States.

Price: Not available

Side Effects: In Phase II clinical trials (published in *Urology* in 2002 and *International Journal of Impotence Research* in 2003), the most common reported side effect was pain at the application site; the majority of reports indicated short-duration, mild to moderate pain. Hypotension (low blood pressure) was an uncommon occurrence, and its incidence was lower than that seen with intra-urethral alprostadil. Large Phase III trials presented at two erectile dysfunction meetings showed no hypotension at 200 and 300 mcg dosages.

Comments: The product is in various stages of clinical testing throughout the world. In double-blind, placebo-controlled Phase III, multicenter, clinical studies conducted in China, the product had an overall efficacy rate of 75 percent with minimal side effects.

Clinical studies have shown that the product works within 15–20 minutes after application, but it could be applied up to one hour before intercourse, making it a versatile product. No significant spousal side effects have been reported with Alprox-TD®.

NexMed is also developing a female version of the drug, Femprox. Phase I trials have been satisfactorily completed. Although Phase II trials are still in the early stages, one has been completed and published (*Journal of Sex and Marital Therapy*, 2001 and 2003). Results of this trial showed a dose-dependent trend of increased sexual arousal.

For more information: 609-208-9688

Web site: *www.nexmedinc.com*

Intraurethral medication

Intraurethral medication consists of drugs that are inserted directly into the urethra through the opening in the penis. One intraurethral medication, MUSE®, is currently available.

MUSE® (Medicated Urethral System for Erection) is a suppository medication in the form of a tiny cylindrical pellet, which is inserted into the penis with a penile syringe. This tubelike device enables the user to place the suppository far enough into the penis for it to take effect. Erections occur in about fifteen minutes.

Urethral Suppository

• MUSE® (alprostadil)   Vivus

Manufacturer: Vivus, Inc.

Brand Name: MUSE®

Active Chemical: Alprostadil

Dosage: Four dosage levels: 125, 250, 500, and 1000 µg

Administration: The medication, in the form of a pellet, is delivered to the urethral membrane by an applicator, which is inserted into the opening of the penis. The man should urinate immediately prior to insertion. The few drops of urine remaining in the urethra lubricate the urinary tract in the penis and make it easier to insert the stem of the MUSE® applicator. Do not use Vaseline or any type of oil or grease as a lubricant because it may interfere with the absorption of the pellet. The first treatment should be under medical supervision.

To minimize or eliminate pain, the penis should be pulled out and upward in order to straighten the urethra prior to inserting the stem of the applicator. The applicator should be inserted slowly and carefully, and withdrawn if resistance is felt. The man should try to insert the applicator again after further straightening the penis. The man is cautioned to insert the applicator slowly.

Status: Available

Price: $115–$140 (price varies with the dose strength prescribed) per box of six doses, 80–85 percent covered by insurance

Side Effects: Intraurethral administration may be psychologically easier than injection. The most common side effect is penile pain, which is due to the effects of the alprostadil being inserted. About one-third of the men in the clinical trial experienced penile pain. Discomfort gradually decreased after multiple administrations.

Comments: Since MUSE® is administered directly into the penis there are no systemic side effects, and since the drug is deposited into the urethra, there is no risk of fibrosis. The erection occurs within 5–10 minutes, allowing for spontaneity. MUSE® may be taken up to twice in a 24-hour period.

A man who fails to respond to injectable medication may still find MUSE® effective. One study reported that 58 percent of the patients who did not respond to injections "achieved an erection satisfactory for intercourse after MUSE® in the clinic, and 50 percent of these responsive patients continued to use MUSE® ... successfully for intercourse at home" (*International Journal of Impotence Research* 8(3):146, 1996). Studies in men with erectile dysfunction as a result of radical prostatectomy showed a success rate of greater than 40 percent.

One physician said that he routinely begins his patients at 500 μg at home, increasing to 1,000 μg if the erection response is insufficient. Men considering using MUSE® should not become dejected if it does not work. As noted previously, no medication will work on everyone.

Vivus reported the effectiveness of intraurethral alprostadil in combination with other vasoactive agents. In one small study, patients were treated with combination therapy of sildenafil and MUSE®. Each medication was administered as usual (i.e., sildenafil was taken 1–1¹/₂ hours before anticipated intercourse) and MUSE® was administered about 10 minutes before. All patients involved reported satisfactory erections after 30 months of combination therapy. In another study using the same drug combination 92 percent of patients treated responded successfully.

Although MUSE® may get blood into the penis to cause an erection, the erection can be maintained only if the blood remains in the penis. Many patients with erectile dysfunction also have an associated disorder of the venoocclusive mechanism called venous leak syndrome. This condition results in the failure to retain blood within the penis. Venous leakage prevents the storage of blood and therefore an erection cannot be maintained. In July 1997, Vivus introduced a venous flow controller, Actis®, which is the only approved adjustable band for use with MUSE®. It is placed at the base of the penis for treatment of venous leak syndrome. The product works to diminish absorption of the alprostadil into the body and to enhance the erectile effect of MUSE® by retaining more alprostadil in the penis and preventing blood from flowing out of the penis. The use of MUSE® plus Actis® is currently under clinical investigation in the United States. In August 1998, Vivus presented research data on the efficacy of MUSE® when used together with Actis®, showing that, during home treatment, 75 percent of administrations of the combination resulted in sexual intercourse.

Erections lasted approximately 25 minutes. The average study patient had moderate to complete erectile dysfunction.

Some men with penile implants have used MUSE® to provide engorgement of the glans (the head of the penis). Engorgement of the glans occurs during natural erections, but not with an implant. Do not do this without first consulting with your doctor.

For more information: 888-367-6873

Web site: *www.vivus.com*

Penile injection (intracavernosal injection)

Most of the work that led to injections began in the late 1980s with Robert Virag's studies on the effect of papaverine. The results were such that by the end of 1998 at least six injection products and compounds were available. This array enabled physicians to address the needs of patients as they concerned effectiveness, penile pain, and other side effects.

A key precondition for using any injectable medication is that the man must be willing to insert a needle into his penis. Most men find that the biggest problem with the needle is the apprehension leading up to its use. Many men feel queasy. However, when the needle is inserted correctly and quickly, a man should feel no more than a nanosecond pinprick in the skin of the penis, much like pinching his earlobe or the skin on his elbow. Some men have found it acceptable for their partner to administer the injection.

Although injection works without stimulation, the penis will be more rigid with stimulation. Key benefits of injection are:

• The erection occurs within five to fifteen minutes.
• The man will have increased stamina and sustainability.
• It is highly effective—injection produces an erection in most cases.

The primary disadvantage is penile pain from the injection and from the medication, experienced by about thirty-seven percent of the men in one clinical trial. In addition, in less than ten percent of men, injection medication can lead to fibrosis (scar tissue) that impairs the delivery of blood to the penis, which worsens erectile dysfunction.

Injection therapy demands close doctor–patient cooperation. The doctor must:

1. Determine the dosage by beginning with an initial dose and observing the effect. This must be done in the physician's office.

2. Ensure that you are properly trained in administering the injection.

The correct technique for the injection requires the medication to be injected in the area of the penis so that the erection will occur and without injury to the vascular part of the penis. Since each man's situation may be different, specific instructions should be obtained from the doctor. Some companies also provide detailed instructions for injections.

a. The head of the penis should be pulled out straight. Looking at the penis from the front, the needle should be inserted at the ten or the two o'clock position nearer to the base rather than the head. If people find it easier to inject the needle straight down instead of at an angle, the penis may be rotated slightly.

b. After the medication is injected, pressure *must* be applied at the injection site for five minutes after the injection. The purpose is to control deep internal bleeding, not surface bleeding. Most of the time (at least eighty percent), skin blood vessels will not be hit, but almost all the time a deep blood vessel will be hit and bleed. (Watch the clock to make sure you really put pressure on the spot for this amount of time; if you try to estimate when five minutes have passed, you will probably not hold the pressure long enough.) This is to prevent blood from collecting deep in the tissue at the spot where the injection was made. If such a collection of blood (hematoma) occurs, it can potentially lead to plaque formation and scar tissue, which can subsequently lead to even more severe erectile dysfunction.

3. Observe that there are no severe complications and address any complications that occur. The doctor's objective is to make sure that you are able to do penile injections at home safely and with the desired effect.

An injection can have serious side effects if the erection lasts too long (greater than four hours). This condition, called priapism, is very painful, and if it is not treated promptly may result in severe tissue damage and permanent loss of potency. If the injection is done properly, a priapism should be a rare event. Caverject® labeling, approved by the FDA, specifies that erections lasting four hours or longer should be treated. The man should seek immediate treatment if an erection lasts four hours. The medication required to end the erection is similar to that used for asthma or high blood pressure. As a precautionary measure, men using injections are advised to have a medication at hand such as phenylephrine, ephedrine, norepinephrine, or epinephrine. Since these medications require a prescription, they should only be obtained from a physician and used according to his or her instructions. Some doctors also suggest taking an over-the-counter decongestant such as pseudoephedrine (Sudafed or many other brands); this treatment should be tried only if the priapism has lasted less than four hours. Before taking any over-the-counter products, as well as any other medications, patients should consult their physician.

This section covers three penile injection products and three blends that doctors may prescribe for particular erectile dysfunction cases.

Men who experience pain with brand name injection medication should be aware that the pain is due primarily to the prostaglandin E-1 (alprostadil). The pain results from the way the prostaglandin is absorbed through the membrane. About fifty percent of the users experience some degree of ache or pain; only ten to twenty percent have severe pain. We know of a doctor who prescribes lidocaine with the injection medication to lessen and in some cases eliminate the pain.

One commercially manufactured injection, Invicorp™, mode by Senetek, does not contain prostaglandin and pain is reported by only about one-tenth of one percent of users. This product is not currently available in the United States.

It is also the prostaglandin component of the tri- and quad-mixes is responsible for most of the pain reported by patients using these formulations. Papaverine, which is a component of all the mixes, can cause penile scarring and requires that the patient have regular liver function tests. Anyone using custom mixes must be monitored by a physician.

For some patients, combinations of active ingredients have been responsible for better erectile responses than any ingredient alone. These combinations are shown at the end of this section. A *World of Urology* 1997 article noted response rates in studies that exceeded ninety percent. One study using a four-drug combination in ninety-four patients resulted in a response rate of ninety-six percent. Any man considering taking any injection medication should explore with his doctor the prospective downsides. Some discomfort accompanies all injections.

Elsewhere in the book we have talked about lifestyle and disease affecting blood vessels in the body so that injections do not work very well. Many other reasons a high number of men discontinue treatment were already noted in Chapter 1. However, reasons that men specifically discontinue injections, otherwise known as intracavernosal therapy, include pain and squeamishness about inserting a needle into the penis.

INJECTABLE (INTRACAVERNOSAL)

- Caverject® (alprostadil)   Pfizer
- EDEX® (alprostadil)   Schwarz Pharma
- Invicorp™   Senetek
  (vasoactive intestinal polypeptide plus phentolamine mesylate)
- Custom combination products
  Bi-mix
  Tri-mix
  Quad-mix

Manufacturer: Pfizer (formerly Pharmacia-Upjohn)

Brand Name: Caverject®

Active Chemical: Alprostadil

Dosage: Caverject Impulse Dual Chamber System 10 µg and 20 µg

Administration: The medication should not be used more than three times a week. Men must allow at least 24 hours to elapse between successive injections.

Following the instructions provided with the system, the user first mixes the liquid and powder by turning the plunger on the syringe. Then the appropriate dose is selected by turning the plunger until the correct dose is shown in a window on the syringe. The technique for administration is safe with proper training. First-time users must be taught how to administer injections by a doctor or qualified health professional. As noted previously, the patient and doctor must work together to determine the appropriate dosage.

Status: Available.

Price: Sold in packages, each containing two kits. Estimated cost in the Washington, DC area for the 10 µg system is $48.00 and for the 20 µg system it is $59.00.

Side Effects: The major complaint is penile pain, which is the direct effect of the medication, not the injection. Discomfort is a function of the dosage, and ranges from a dull ache to burning pain. During the clinical trials, the company reports about 37 percent of the patients had penile pain. Severe pain is experienced by 10–20 percent of men. Fibrosis (forming of little nodules in the penis) is a concern.

Comments: According to Pfizer, this medication is indicated when the cause for erectile dysfunction is due to neurological, vascular, or psychological problems, as well as mixed causes. This includes the typical prostate cancer-related causes. It should not be used when the man has conditions that could lead to prolonged erections (priapism). According to one erectile dysfunction specialist, there is less risk of priapism with Caverject® than with other injectables.

Caverject® systems use a superfine 29-gauge needle.

For more information: 800-879-3477

Web site: *www.caverject.com, www.impotent.com*

Manufacturer: Schwarz Pharma

Trade Name: EDEX®

Active Chemical: Alprostadil

Dosage: EDEX® kits and cartridges are supplied in strengths of 10, 20, and 40 µg. The product should not be used more than three times per week and there should be at least 24 hours between each dose. The optimum dosage should be determined for each patient in the doctor's office.

Administration: EDEX® is available in two forms: (1) as a powder that must be mixed with the saline solution provided in a kit and (2) as a cartridge where the solution and powder are in one container. The cartridge is placed in the reusable EDEX® injection device that is used to reconstitute the sterile powder. EDEX® is given as an intracavernous injection over a 5- to 10-second interval. As with all injections, drops or solutions should not be added to the product provided by the manufacturer.

Status: Available. Prescription only. Introduced June 1997.

Price: $120–$135 for four shots of the 20 µg and $169–$185 for four shots of the 40 µg dosage.

Side Effects: About 41 percent of patients had penile pain during the first two months, which decreased over time (3 percent during months 21–24). Some patients experienced prolonged erections. Fibrosis is also a concern.

Comments: EDEX® is indicated for the treatment of erectile dysfunction due to neurological, vascular, psychological, or mixed causes.

EDEX® should not be used in patients who are sensitive to the active chemical alprostadil or any other prostaglandins, or in patients who have conditions that might increase the possibility of priapism (prolonged erection), such as sickle-cell anemia, multiple myeloma, or anatomical deformations of the penis. Patients with penile implants should not be treated with EDEX®.

Schwarz provides 29-gauge needles for use with the cartridges. The company provides a 27-gauge needle and an optional, thinner 30-gauge needle with kits to minimize injection discomfort.

One study compared the efficacy, safety, and patient preference of EDEX® with MUSE® plus optional Actis® tension system. During the in-office titration and at-home phases of the study, EDEX® was more effective than MUSE® in producing erections sufficient for sexual intercourse. Patient satisfaction and preference were also greater with EDEX® than with MUSE®. Another study indicated that EDEX® was effective, based on responses to a questionnaire in 85–89 percent of men who did not respond to sildenafil (Viagra®).

For more information: 800-558-5114, or 262-238-9994

Web site: *www.edex.com*

Manufacturer: Senetek

Trade Name: Invicorp™

Active Chemical: Vasoactive intestinal polypeptide in combination with the adrenergic drug phentolamine mesylate (PMS)

Dosage: Information not available

Administration: Proprietary state-of-the-art autoinjector

Status: Not available in the United States. Available in Denmark and possibly in the United Kingdom (See "Comments.")

Price: Not available

Side Effects: Penile pain during the injection was experienced by about 0.12 percent of the men. Pain after the injection was experienced by 0.013 percent of men. In addition, the medication can lead to fibrosis, which impairs the delivery of blood to the penis.

Comments: In March 1999, the United Kingdom's Committee on Safety of Medicines of the Medicines Control Agency decided to advise the Licensing Authority to authorize the marketing of Senetek's Invicorp™ new drug therapy for treating moderate to severe, organic-based erectile dysfunction. The company expects full marketing authorization. In 1998, the Danish Medicine Agency approved Invicorp™ for the treatment of moderate to severe erectile dysfunction.

In clinical studies published in the March 1999 issue of the *British Journal of Urology*, Invicorp™ proved effective in 82 percent of patients. In another study, the company noted that 59 percent of the patients treated successfully with Invicorp™ "had previously been treated with alternative pharmacotherapies, including prostaglandin, papaverine, and yohimbine but had withdrawn from treatment either due to lack of effectiveness or side effects."

For more information: 800-758-5804

Web site: *www.senetekplc.com*

Manufacturer: Individual doctors prescribing their own mixes

Brand Name: Custom combination products—no brand name because doctors prescribe their own compounds; hence the label "blends."

Active Chemical: Injectable medications come in basic combinations, as well as in what are known as bi-mix, tri-mix, and even quad-mix. Specifically, these combinations are:

Bi-mix: papaverine-phentolamine (better than papaverine alone)

Tri-mix: papaverine-phentolamine-prostaglandin E-1

Quad-mix: forskolin-papaverine-phentolamine-prostaglandin E-1

Dosage: Varies by patient

Administration: Penile injection

Status: Formula determined by local doctor

Price: Pharmacy price is approximately $150–$250 for 20 shots, depending on dosage and combination.

Side Effects: Penile pain, fibrosis

Comments: Penile pain is primarily due to prostaglandin E-1. Doctors are adjusting the prostaglandin portion when patients complain of pain.

Tri-mix: In one study, the tri-mix worked in 62 percent of the patients who had failed to respond to other injections. Some men had penile pain.

Quad-mix: This product was developed for men on whom tri-mix did not work. In one study comparing tri-mix and quad-mix, the inclusion of forskolin in quad-mix "resulted in substantial improvements in rigidity and duration, 47 percent vs. 80 percent rigidity and 20 mins. vs. 67 mins" (*Journal of Urology* 155(5)A743, 996).

For more information: Contact your physician.

New medications in development

The following medications are in development and are not currently available for use. They are included here as an indication of the research that is ongoing in the field of erectile dysfunction treatment. This is by no means a complete listing of potential new products or product types.

The following products are presented in alphabetical order by manufacturer:

• GPI 1485   Guilford Pharmaceuticals
• PT-141   Palatin Technologies

Manufacturer: Guilford Pharmaceuticals

Brand Name: GPI 1485

Active Chemical: Neuroimmunophilin ligand

Dosage: Information not available

Administration: Information not available

Status: In development

Price: Information not available

Side Effects: Information not available

Comments: This product is intended to stimulate regeneration of the nerves. See the section on neural regeneration in this chapter. GPI 1485 belongs to a class of compounds called neuro-immunophilin ligands. Neuroimmunophilin ligands are small molecules that, in preclinical experiments, have been shown to repair and regenerate damaged nerves without affecting normal, healthy nerves. Neuroimmunophilin ligands may have an application in the treatment of peripheral nerve injuries such as post-prostatectomy erectile dysfunction.

GPI 1485 has demonstrated significant neuroprotective and neuroregenerative activity in preclinical models of postprostatec-tomy erectile dysfunction. Guilford Pharmaceuticals is beginning a multicenter, placebo-controlled Phase II clinical study of GPI 1485 in patients undergoing radical prostatectomy for prostate cancer, in order to assess the drug's efficacy in improving erectile dysfunction.

For more information: Company does not wish to be contacted while the drug is under FDA review.

Web site: *www.guilfordpharm.com*

Manufacturer: Palatin Technologies

Brand Name: PT-141

Active Chemical: Melanocortin agonist

Dosage: Information not available

Administration: Intranasal (nasal spray)

Status: In development

Price: Information not available

Side Effects: Information not available

Comments: PT-141 works by activating neurons in the area of the brain responsible for sexual function.

A Phase IIB clinical trial in men with erectile dysfunction was completed in September 2003, and the results were reported at a conference in Los Angeles, California in November 2003. In the trial, there was statistically significant improvement in erections in all the dosing levels tested. No cardiovascular side effects were observed. According to a Reuters news release in November 2003, the earliest approval for this class of drug would be late 2007 or early 2008.

For more information: 609-495-2200

Web site: *www.palatin.com*

Devices

Three types of devices are discussed here: penile splints, vacuum erection devices, and penile implants, also called prostheses. Vacuum erection devices and penile splints are generally considered noninvasive, although some doctors consider vacuum therapy as minimally invasive. Penile implants require major surgery but once in place they are unobtrusive, and do not require extensive preparation for use.

Penile splints and supports. A support is basically a penile splint that supports the penis in penetration. These splints have been available in adult stores for a long time.

In 1996, American MedTech introduced its first product, a penile support sleeve called Rejoyn. This is a variant of the old penile splint. The company's material states: "Rejoyn is designed to enable a man with a flaccid penis to engage in intercourse."

Rejoyn is a "patented penile support sleeve ... made of high grade, natural feeling Santoprene (neoprene) rubber" that fits around the penis. The support sleeve is held in place by a strap that wraps behind the scrotum and which is designed to break away for easy removal. A lubricated Comfort Cover is then placed over the sleeve; these covers resemble a condom with a hole in the front, and may be pulled back to expose the head of the penis to allow for greater sensation for both partners. The stiffness of the neoprene provides the support. We've been told that the woman needs to control movement; otherwise, the penile support could hurt her.

For further information, call Rejoyn at 800-578-6916 or visit their Web site at *www.rejoyn.com*.

Vacuum therapy systems. The first medical vacuum device for treating erectile dysfunction was initially developed in the 1960s by Geddings Osbon in Augusta, Georgia. This became commercially available in 1984. Currently there are estimated to be over two million users of vacuum erection devices worldwide. Doctors frequently prescribe them because they are relatively safe and noninvasive, provide immediate results, and have a high rate of success.

This type of device creates a vacuum around the penis using a negative pressure device (sometimes referred to as a vacuum device or pump); this vacuum causes blood to flow into the penile tissues, thus creating an erection. Vacuum therapy systems consist of a cylinder (the vacuum chamber), vacuum pump (manual or battery-operated), tension rings (also called tension systems or support rings), and water-based lubricant. The steps for using a vacuum pump are as follows:

1. Connect the negative pressure device to the cylinder.
2. Lubricate the penis and place it inside the cylinder.
3. Position the cylinder firmly against the body to form an air-tight seal.
4. Activate the negative pressure device to remove air from the cylinder. This creates negative pressure inside the cylinder and causes blood to be drawn into the penis to create an erection.
5. A tension ring is then placed at the base of the penis to maintain the erection. If a tension system is not used, the blood will flow back into the body and the erection will be lost.

There are some differences between a natural erection and one created by a vacuum therapy system:

- The penis may become "cool" after a short period because the constriction ring decreases blood flow into the penis, as well as maintaining the erection by preventing blood flow out of the penis.
- The penis may be bigger around and longer than with a natural erection because the tissues of the penis beyond the tension ring are distended with blood; this distension results in the rigidity and tumescence of the erection. (During a natural erection the entire vascular system of the penis, which extends from within the body to the glans, is engorged.) The penis may appear darker, and the veins will stand out.
- There may be little vertical control of the penis. The penis may pivot at the base because it is rigid only beyond the tension ring. In a natural erection, hardness extends back into the body. However, after penetration has been accomplished, the "pivot

effect" or the "hinge effect" as it is sometimes called, does not interfere with intercourse.

Several sexual dysfunction specialists noted that erectile success with a vacuum therapy system is about ninety-eight percent, though a common complaint is that vacuum systems are a lot of fuss. However, bear in mind that vacuum therapy has immediate results without the uncertainty and lack of predictability of drug therapy. Despite the foregoing effects, and possibly some loss of sensitivity, long-term satisfaction is about seventy to seventy-five percent. One specialist noted that about half the dropouts go on to implants.

A list of manufacturers and their vacuum systems to treat erectile dysfunction is included at the end of this section.

Caution: One vacuum therapy system is not the same as another. Since use of such systems creates physical and to some extent physiological changes in the penis, you should use a vacuum system only with care and following a consultation with a physician. Erectile dysfunction may be a warning sign for an undiagnosed serious health problems, such as diabetes, high blood pressure, or cancer. Your particular situation may make it advisable to consult a urologist or sexual dysfunction specialist.

Some of the vacuum devices listed here are available without prescription. Nevertheless, Medicare and many private insurance plans continue to reimburse patients for prescribed vacuum therapy systems. If you intend to use a vacuum device, a doctor's prescription should be obtained even if you plan to purchase an over-the-counter model because you may be eligible for reimbursement.

A cautionary note: On September 10, 1997, the FDA issued an Interim Regulatory Policy guideline for external rigidity devices. The guideline specified a maximum safe vacuum limit of seventeen inches of mercury (four hundred forty millimeters of mercury). Make sure that any vacuum device you purchase meets this safety requirement.

Although all vacuum therapy systems operate on the same principles and have many basic features in common, there are differences that may make one model easier or more comfortable to use. This is particularly true of the design of the pump handle (of manual models), the number and size of the adapters provided to achieve the best fit for the penis into the cylinder, and the sizing and design of the tension system rings and their application system. Your partner should be included in the decision of which vacuum system to purchase because you must work together in using this aid. The vacuum therapy systems are described, and listed in alphabetical order by manufacturer.

- Soma Therapy ED Touch® II   Augusta Medical Systems
- Soma Therapy ED Response® II   Augusta Medical Systems
- Soma Therapy ED SomaCorrect™   Augusta Medical Systems
- Soma Therapy ED Prostatectomy
  Recovery Aid™   Augusta Medical Systems
- Vitality Plus™   Augusta Medical Systems
- Vitality™   Augusta Medical Systems
- Assist®   Augusta Medical Systems
- ImpoAid™ VTU-1   Encore Medical Products
- ImpoAid™ Deluxe Rx System   Encore Medical Products
- VED Ultra®   Mission Pharmacal
- VED Classic®   Mission Pharmacal
- Rejoyn Vacuum Therapy System   Pos-T-Vac
- Bos 2000-2   Pos-T-Vac
- IVP-600™   Pos-T-Vac
- MVP-700™   Pos-T-Vac
- ErecAid™ Esteem™ System   Timm Medical Technology
- Vacurect™ Rx   Vacurect Manufacturing (Pty) Ltd.
- Vacurect™ OTC   Vacurect Manufacturing (Pty) Ltd.

Manufacturer: Augusta Medical Systems

Brand Name: SomaTherapy-ED Touch® II

SomaTherapy-ED Response® II

SomaTherapy-ED SomaCorrect™

SomaTherapy-ED Prostatectomy Recovery Aid™

Vitality Plus™

Vitality™

Assist™

Cost: SomaTherapy-ED Touch® II—$548.00

SomaTherapy-ED Response® II—$495.00

SomaTherapy-ED SomaCorrect™—$495.00

SomaTherapy-ED Prostatectomy Recovery Aid™—$495.00

Vitality Plus®—$259.00

Vitality®—$199.00

Assist®—$99.00

Prescription: A prescription is required for the Touch® II, Response® II, SomaCorrect™, and Prostatectomy Recovery Aid™. Vitality™, Vitality Plus™, and Assist™ are available over-the-counter.

Description: The Response® II is a manually operated vacuum therapy system operated by a handle on the side of the negative pressure device (pump head), which is operated by squeezing the handle against the side of the negative pressure device. The system includes two adapters, a loading cone, and two different-sized SureRelease™ single-use support rings (three in each size).

The Touch® II is a batter-operated vacuum therapy system, which also includes two adapters, a loading cone, and two different-sized SureRelease™ single-use support rings.

Vitality Plus™, Vitality™, and Assist™ are, respectively, battery and manual, nonprescription vacuum therapy systems.

The Prostatectomy Recovery Aid™ is a vacuum system designed for patients undergoing prostatectomy. It should be prescribed prior to the patient's surgery so that he can become proficient and comfortable using the device ahead of time.

The Soma Correct System is intended for the treatment of Peyronie's disease and consists of a manual vacuum therapy system and three variably sized cylinders.

Comments: Augusta Medical Systems provides 24-hour, 7-day-a-week Toll-Free Technical Support for both patients and prescribing physicians and a field staff that meets privately with patients in the physician's office or clinic to support the use of SomaTherapy-ED by providing actual application training and problem resolution. The company also has a buy-back program if the system fails to produce a quality erection for the patient, if the patient meets certain criteria (see the literature included with products).

For more information: 800-827-8382

Web site: *www.augustams.com*

Manufacturer: Encore Medical Products

Brand Name: ImpoAid™ VTU-1

ImpoAid™ VTU-E

ImpoAid™ Deluxe Rx System

Cost: VTU-1—$129.95 (MSRP)

VTU-E—$169.95 (MSRP)

Deluxe—$400.00 (MSRP)

ImpoAid Ring Assortment—$29.95

Prescription: No prescription is required for the VTU-1 and VTU-E. The Deluxe system is covered by Medicare with a doctor's prescription.

Description: The VTU-1 is a manually operated vacuum therapy system; the pump handle is in line with the penile tube (vacuum chamber). It includes seven different-sized constriction rings. There is a lifetime warranty on the pump and tube. Instruction manual and video are included. The VTU-E is a battery-operated model.

The Deluxe System has a battery-operated pump and also includes a manual pump. Seven different-sized constriction rings are included. The system comes in a zippered carrying case and includes a video and a lifetime warranty.

Comments: Encore has a toll-free help line.

For more information: 800-221-6603

Web site: *www.impoaid.com*

Manufacturer: Mission Pharmacal

Brand Name: VED Ultra®

                           VED Classic®

Cost: VED Ultra®—$125.00

                 VED Classic®—$115.00

Prescription: No prescription is required. However, cost may be covered by Medicare with a physician's prescription.

Description: The VED Ultra® is a battery-operated model.

The VED Classic® is a manual vacuum therapy system. The pump is a separate unit attached to the penile cylinder with plastic tubing.

Comments: No charge for shipping. There is a two-year warranty on vacuum pump and cylinder.

For more information: 877-833-8587

Web site: *www.missionnpharmacal.com*

Manufacturer: Pos-T-Vac

Brand Name: Rejoyn Vacuum Therapy System

Bos 2000-2

IVP-600™

MVP-700™

Cost: Rejoyn—$129.85

Bos 2000-2—$169.85

IVP-600™—$129.00

MVP-700™—$350.00

Prescription: No prescription is required. However, the cost may be covered by Medicare with a physician's prescription.

Description: The Rejoyn is a manual vacuum therapy system, with a plunger-type pump handle, which is offset to one side. Vacuum is created by the push-pull action of the pump handle. The system includes four different-sized support rings, a ring-loading cone to facilitate putting the ring on the tube, and an adapter bushing used to fit the tube to the penis.

The IVP-600™ is a manual system; the pump head is in line with the penile tube and the vacuum is created by compressing the pump head toward the body. This system includes two adapter bushings, a ring loading cone, and three different-sized support rings.

The MVP-700™ is a manual pump, with a plunger-type pump handle, which is offset to one side. The system includes three adapter bushings, a ring loading cone, and four different-sized support rings.

The Bos 2000-2 is a battery-operated pump; one adapter bushing, a ring loading cone, and three different sizes of support rings are included with purchase.

For more information: 800-279-7434

Web site: *www.postvac.com*

Manufacturer: TIMM Medical Technologies (a subsidiary of Endocare, Inc.)

Brand Name: ErecAid™ Esteem™ System

Cost: $395.00 and up (figures from Internet sites)

Prescription: A prescription is required.

Description: The ErecAid™ Esteem™ System consists of a negative pressure device (either manually or battery-operated) and a cylinder that attaches to the pump at one end, then fits over the penis and is held snugly against the body to create a vacuum seal. The manual model is operated by a squeeze action of the lever-type handle. To maintain the erection, Pressure-Point™ Tension rings are used; four rings are included with each system. To facilitate placement of the rings onto the cylinder an Easy Action™ Ring Applicator is also included.

Comments: There is a 90-day return policy on systems purchased directly from Endocare, with a refund of either 100 percent or 50 percent of the suggested retail price, depending on compliance with policy (detailed in instruction manual).

For more information: 1-800-346-7266

Web site: *www.timmmedical.com*

Manufacturer: Vacurect Manufacturing (Pty) Ltd.

Distributor: Bonro Medical Inc.

Brand Name: Vacurect™ Rx

Vacurect™ OTC

Cost: Vacurect™ Rx $465.00

Vacurect™ OTC $179.00

Prescription: The Vacurect™ Rx requires a prescription. The Vacurect™ OTC is available as an over-the-counter model.

Description: Both Vacurect™ models are manually operated. Ten different-sized tension systems, which are reusable, are included. The unique design of this device integrates the negative pressure actuating mechanism (pump) and the penile cylinder (vacuum chamber) into a compact one-piece unit. The pumping action, which creates the vacuum, is accomplished by means of a pump sleeve that slides up and down over the cylinder. The tension ring fits *inside* the cylinder at the end that is toward the body, so no special applicator is required to fit the ring onto the cylinder. Initially the cylinder is placed only over the head of the penis, and the pumping action draws the penis into the cylinder as the erection is created by the vacuum, until the cylinder is against the body. Once the erection has been achieved, the vacuum inside the cylinder is released leaving the tension ring in place at the base of the penis to maintain the erection.

The Vacurect™ systems include the vacuum unit, travel pouch, ten different-sized tension systems, service oil (to lubricate the pump), personal lubricant, and instructions.

Comments: Free shipping via USPS Priority Mail for either model. These products are covered by a three-year replacement warranty on the vacuum unit. The product also carries a 30-day 80 percent money back satisfaction guarantee.

Bonro Medical, Inc. provides 24-hour, 7-day-a-week toll-free technical support for both patients and physicians.

For more information: 866-692-6676

Web site: *www.bonro.com; www.vacurect.com*

Penile implants. A penile implant is a mechanical device that enables an erection. It is surgically implanted into the penis to permit the user to have an erection at will. Implants were more widely recommended as the solution of choice for erectile dysfunction prior to the introduction of injections and oral medications. Many men choose this procedure when available medication is not effective.

Implants can last eight to twenty years. Some implant procedures are performed as minor outpatient surgery. However, all surgery carries certain risks, which should be thoroughly discussed with the doctor. These include postoperative infection, pain, and device malfunction. One prostate cancer survivor reported that surgery for a semirigid prosthesis required a two-day hospital stay. He noted it was *"tough* surgery. Recovery was longer than for my radical prostatectomy."

There are three forms of implants:

1. *Semirigid-malleable:* Consisting of wire bundles enclosed in a silicon shaft, it is "worn" bent down and straightened for intercourse.
   Advantages:
   This implant is a simple device and not likely to fail for mechanical reasons.
   May be the best choice for men with limited manual dexterity.
   Easy to use.
   Simplest surgical procedure for placement.
   Least expensive.
   Disadvantages:
   The implant is rigid all the time and is not cosmetically natural, although it is not usually noticeable under most types of clothing.
   The penis may not feel as natural when erect or flaccid.
2. *Inflatable:* The two most common types are referred to as two-piece and three-piece. The two-piece prostheses consist of implantable cylinders placed in the corpora cavernosa and a pump that is placed in the scrotum. The inflation of the cylinders causes the erection and is accomplished by means of saline solution. The reservoirs for the saline are actually in the pump or the cylinders depending on the implant type. The three-piece prostheses are composed of two cylinders implanted in the corpora cavernosa, a pump placed in the scrotum, and a reservoir placed in the abdomen; tubing connects all the parts.

Advantages of the two-piece type:
More easily concealed than a malleable implant.
Small, easy-to-use inflation pump.
Fast, easy, one-step deflation procedure.
Fewer components than a three-piece type.
Disadvantages:
Requires some manual dexterity to operate pump.
Possibility of leakage, clog, or device malfunction.
Contains more mechanical components than a malleable device.
Advantages of the three-piece system:
Feels most like a natural erection.
Feels more firm and full than other prostheses; cylinders on some models expand in girth, as well as length.
When deflated, is softer and feels more flaccid than other prostheses, and is most easily concealed under clothing.
Disadvantages:
Requires some manual dexterity to operate the pump.
Contains more mechanical components than other prostheses.
Possibility of leakage, clog, or device malfunction.
Possibility of inadvertent erections.
Most expensive.

The devices are described in this section alphabetically by manufacturer:

• AMS 700 CX™ / CXR™ Inflatable Penile Prosthesis	American Medical Systems
• AMS 700 Ultrex™ Inflatable Penile Prosthesis	American Medical Systems
• AMS Ambicor®	American Medical Systems
• AMS DURA II™	American Medical Systems
• AMS Malleable 600M™ / 650M™	American Medical Systems
• Alpha 1® Inflatable Penile Prosthesis	Mentor
• Titan™ Inflatable Penile Prosthesis	Mentor
• Acu-Form® Penile Prosthesis	Mentor

Manufacturer: American Medical Systems

Brand Names: AMS 700 CX™ / CXR™ Inflatable Penile Prosthesis

AMS 700 Ultrex™ Inflatable Penile Prosthesis

AMS Ambicor®

AMS DURA II™

AMS Malleable® 600M™ / 650M™ (in Europe)

Description: *AMS 700 Product Line:* These prostheses are generally described as three-piece inflatable prostheses. They are composed of two cylinders that are implanted in the corpora cavernosa, a reservoir, and a pump; the parts are connected by tubing. The reservoir is placed into the lower abdomen, and the pump is placed into the scrotum. The pump is used to both inflate and deflate the cylinders. The 700 CX and CXR expand in width only; the 700 Ultrex expands in both length and width.

AMS Ambicor®: This is a two-piece inflatable prosthesis. It consists of two cylinders that are implanted in the corpora cavernosa, and a pump placed in the scrotum. Within each cylinder is a reservoir of fluid; when the pump is activated, the fluid is moved from the reservoir area into the main body of the cylinders, thus creating an erection. To return the penis to the flaccid state, pressure on the cylinders will move the fluid back into the reservoirs.

AMS DURA II™ and Malleable®: These prostheses are composed of two rods made of wire bundles and covered with polyester yarn inside a solid silicone elastomer casing. One rod is placed in each corpus cavernosum. The rods are straightened for intercourse, and bent downward around the scrotum for concealment.

Comments

For more information: 800-328-3881

Web site: *www.visitams.com*

Manufacturer: Mentor

Brand Names: Alpha I® Inflatable Penile Prosthesis

Titan™ Inflatable Penile Prosthesis

Acu-Form® Penile Prosthesis

Description: The Alpha I® and Titan™ are three-piece inflatable implants, consisting of two inflatable cylinders that are implanted in the corpora, a pump placed in the scrotum, and a reservoir, which is placed in the lower abdomen; the parts are connected with tubing.

The Acu-Form is a malleable prosthesis that is used in pairs; one prosthesis is inserted in each corpus cavernosum. Each prosthesis is made of flexible silicone elastomer, with a silver wire coil and a silver helix in the flexible center section. One end of each prosthesis is trimmable to provide appropriate individualized fit. The rods are straightened for intercourse, and bent downward around the scrotum for concealment.

For more information: 800-525-0245

Web site: *www.mentorcorp.com*

Surgery

Neural therapies. This section is particularly important for men who have been diagnosed with, *but have not yet undergone treatment for,* prostate cancer or any cancer that will require pelvic surgery that may compromise the neurovascular bundles responsible for retaining potency. The following techniques are used to try to preserve or regain the maximum possible erectile capability. Men and their partners should ask their doctors the questions listed at the end of this section.

This section discusses nerve sparing and nerve grafting surgical techniques, as well as neural regeneration. They all seek to retain neural capability for obtaining erections. The first two approaches are currently available for appropriate patients. Neural regeneration is being researched and in clinical trials.

Erections were considered a lost capability when men had radical prostatectomy surgery until Dr. Patrick Walsh developed his nerve sparing technique for this procedure, which may be also applicable for other pelvic surgeries. Patients and health care professionals initially considered the technique a "magic bullet" for men needing the surgery. Consequently, men who expected that their surgeons would use this technique were disappointed when they could not achieve erections.

Not only has Dr. Walsh opened the doorway to capability for many men but his work, begun in the late 1980s, has been a catalyst for researchers and companies to look for other ways to retain and rebuild the neural network critical for erectile function. About a decade after the onset of nerve sparing surgery, that technique was followed by nerve grafting surgery, and by the beginning of the twenty-first century, research had commenced on neural regeneration.

Nerve sparing surgery. Dr. Walsh's nerve sparing technique is usually thought of as surgery but in reality it is an avoidance technique used during surgery. Dr. Walsh's technique allows surgeons to use their skill to avoid cutting nerves when removing diseased prostates, if at all possible. Unfortunately, the technique is not suitable in some cases because the surgeon sees that the disease has spread outside the prostate. Also, the technique is not a sure thing because a nerve consists of many tiny fibers spread out in the tissue and is not like a large cable that is easily seen and can be easily avoided. A man's internal anatomy really decides how easy it will be for the surgeon to find the strands of nerves. Some may be spared while others will be cut even though the intent is to keep all of them intact.

As stated above, the nerve bundle is not like a big cable that can be easily seen. Surgeons know generally where the nerves are located. Although they are an "average of 4.9 millimeters away from the prostate" Dr. Stephen Strum writes, in *A Primer on Prostate Cancer*, they can range from 3.2 to 9.5 millimeters. At best, the surgeon can see only some strands of nerve fibers. It is extremely unlikely that all the nerves needed for one hundred percent potency will be preserved because they cannot be seen.

However, doctors now have a tool to confirm the location of the cavernous nerves. In 1997, the FDA approved marketing of a new device. Cavermap, a hand-held device with a nerve stimulator at its end is used during surgery. A ring is fastened around the penis. When the probe is held against a nerve, the ring measures the swelling of the penis from the increased or decreased blood flow that would affect an erection, thereby locating the cavernous nerves. The device has become even more valuable since 2000, when neural grafting was introduced.

Several studies have noted that a significant percentage of patients on whom the device was used to locate the nerves recover erectile function. Dr. Arthur Burnett's overview paper, "Strategies to Promote Recovery of Cavernous Nerve Function after Radical Prostatectomy," cites a study that "erections were better in the Cavermap-assisted group than in the group in which the tool was not used." However, he also notes other studies with conflicting results "dampen enthusiasm for the practical role of this tool at this time either to assist in performing nerve-sparing surgery or to predict erectile function recover afterwards." Also, using the CaverMap may increase the cost of the surgery and increase time for the procedure.

There is a third factor that has an impact on the success rate: age. The younger the man, the better function he will generally have before surgery. Since he has more capability to begin with, he will probably have more after the procedure. In addition, younger people usually recover much more quickly from traumatic events, whether injury or surgery. As men get into their sixties, erectile capability may take up to two years to return. Dr. Walsh contends that, if the surgery is done correctly on men for whom the procedure is appropriate, at least sixty percent of patients who have nerve sparing surgery are completely potent, that is, they should have normal sexual function after surgery. It should be noted that Dr. Walsh operates mostly on younger, healthier men; so a sixty percent success rate is not a realistic expectation for the average prostate cancer patient.

Surgical competence is also a key factor in the surgery's success rate. A man contemplating nerve sparing surgery should make sure that the surgeon does these procedures frequently and in volume. Many surgeons will say, to maintain currency in any technique, a practitioner must do at least one or two each week. Doing the procedures continually is important because skill is refined and technique is reinforced.

Dr. Christopher J. Logothetis, M.D., Chairman of the Department of Genitourinary Medical Oncology, M.D. Anderson Cancer Center, Houston, noted that the technique is practiced "with variable skill at many cancer centers." He goes on to say:

> Although the operation has been widely applied, the elements that contribute to its success are as follows:
> - Adequate initial pathologic assessment and clinical staging, which lead to the proper selection of patients.
> - A "fit" and motivated patient who does not have other medical factors contributing to impotence.
> In a motivated patient who is correctly selected, a nerve-sparing prostatectomy can result in a cure of the cancer and avoid impotence in a number of cases. However, nerve sparing prostatectomy may not be the correct operation in all circumstances because of the following:
> - The location of the cancer does not permit a nerve sparing approach without an excessive risk of incompletely removing the cancer.
> - The cancer is too high-grade or extensive to consider a curative operation.

Even though the nerve sparing technique is widely used, the point regarding surgeon competence must be taken seriously.

Seven questions should be asked of any surgeon you are considering to do your procedure. This is part of managing your health. If the doctor refuses to answer them, you might ask your family doctor to ask the surgeon or possibly consider another practitioner.

1. *Are you a candidate for nerve sparing surgery?* The answer relates to staging of your disease, your medical health, and your level of erectile capability before treatment.

2. *Does the surgeon do nerve sparing prostatectomy?* Some doctors are clear in that they say they take a broad swath of tissue to increase the probability of getting as much disease as possible.

3. *How did the surgeon learn the technique?* As with any new procedure or technique, doctors must be educated and trained. Disseminating clinical knowledge and, more importantly, critical and delicate surgical technique takes years.

4. *For what period of time has the surgeon been doing nerve sparing prostatectomies?* You do not want to be part of a surgeon's learning curve.

5. *How many procedures does the surgeon do monthly?* The answer is an indication of proficiency. The minimum should be four for the surgeon to retain and improve the skill.

6. *Will the surgeon give you the names of patients on whom he or she performed prostatectomies?*

7. *You can also ask the surgeon about the percentage of patients that have regained their potency.* Ask about the percentage of patients who are totally impotent and the percentage capable of achieving intercourse.

Nerve grafting surgery. When sural nerve grafting as a treatment for erectile dysfunction became a reality in 2000, it appeared to be an apparent alternative for patients to retain potency in cases where the nerves responsible for erections must be cut. However, nerve grafting may not hold real promise for most men. *This procedure must be done at the time of the initial surgery; it is not an option for men who have already had a prostatectomy.*

After prostatectomy, there is no way to locate the tiny fibers that make up the cavernous nerves because they are obscured by scar tissue from the initial surgery, and because they "withered away" (atrophied) from lack of stimulation. The same issues that are relevant for preserving the neurovascular bundles also apply here: the extent of the disease, the patient's medical health, and the preoperative level of potency.

Pioneered by Dr. Edward Kim at the University of Tennessee and Dr. Peter Scardino, Memorial Sloan-Kettering Cancer Center, this technique uses the sural nerve (taken from the ankle) to form a connection between the ends of the cavernosal nerves when they must be cut during radical prostatectomy. Whether it is the sural nerve (the section behind the long, straight nerve that runs from the calf down to the ankle) or the newer approach of taking the ilio-inguinal nerve (which is in the lower part of the abdomen), it is sewn to the two ends of the cavernous nerve.

The grafted pieces cannot transmit the nerve signals from one end of the cavernous nerve to the other. They serve as bridges so that the ends of the cavernous nerve can grow toward each other and reconnect. The cavernous nerves are slow growing, about one millimeter a day. At that rate it will take about three and a half weeks to grow an inch. Recovering cavernous nerve function may take several years depending on the length of the gap between the ends of the nerves.

Early estimates of effectiveness ranging from twenty-five to forty-three percent have prompted surgeons to adopt nerve grafting as a primary means for preserving potency in men where one or both cavernous nerves must be cut in the course of a radical prostatectomy. Grafting may never become one hundred percent effective because there is no one cavernosal nerve; it is a complex of fibers distributed in the tissue along the blood vessels to form the neurovascular bundle. It is more like a bundle of wires or lengths of string that are imbedded in the tissue. So the grafting really is placing the section to be grafted so that the maximum number of fibers can be connected. It is a means for improving the recovery of erectile function, not an assurance that recovery will be one hundred percent.

Nerves heal very slowly, and recovering the transmission function could take years. Be aware that, in reported studies, younger men were used, and all had good function prior to surgery. As may be expected, additional surgery is required to obtain and attach the nerve segment. Neural grafting requires longer surgery times and requires a plastic surgeon as well, because the sural nerve is taken from the ankle, and of course the total cost is higher.

Now that the way has been shown, other surgeons are experimenting with grafting other nerves in place, such as the ilio-inguinal nerve. But before this is seen as the solution to surgically caused impotence, Dr. Arthur Burnett offers several cautions. In his overview, he quotes results as:

> showing graft replacement in the setting recovered erections to a level better than without (78 percent vs. 30 percent) and approximating the results of bi-lateral nerve-sparing surgery (79 percent).

> [Although] These demonstrations support the potential value of cavernous interpositions grafting for restoring erectile function in men undergoing radical prostatectomy ... enthusiasm for this sort of intervention should be restrained until indications are defined for the appropriate use of nerve grafts to replace resected cavernous nerves.

His other argument is that men whose cavernous nerves must be cut are not likely to have organ-confined disease, therefore other treatments they may need after surgery, such as radiation or hormone treatment, could counter the benefits of the graft.

Neural regeneration. Another approach to retaining some degree of potency has entered development. But here too considerations to be kept in mind are whether men will really benefit from the new medical technology. One company is known to be researching and developing a compound that could be administered before and after surgery to promote healing of the nerves. In preclinical experiments, Guilford Pharmaceuticals has shown that small molecules called neuroimmunophilin ligands appear to have the capability to repair and regenerate damaged nerves without affecting normal, healthy nerves. Since this is not a surgical approach, a detailed write-up is provided in the "New Medications in Development" section in this chapter (page 144).

Penile vascular surgery. The treatments described here are usually not effective for prostate cancer patients, but are effective for impotence caused by certain injuries.

Two surgical procedures are used to ensure adequate blood in the penis for erection. Vascular surgery in the penis may be used to bypass an obstruction in one of the main penile arteries using a procedure call *penile vascularization.* Alternatively, if the erection cannot be maintained due to venous leakage, a procedure call *venous ligation* may be performed.

Circulation in the penis is complex and the surgery takes about six hours. Complications may include uncontrolled bleeding in the penis during the first few weeks after surgery, pain in the penis, and diminished sensation. In addition, the surgery may cause a shortening of the penis.

According to Dr. Irwin Goldstein, the primary candidates are young men (teenagers to men in their forties) who have suffered an injury. Other criteria used for patient selection for this surgery by Dr. Goldstein include:

• Consistent erectile dysfunction with personal distress.

• No traditional vascular risk factors (hypertension, cigarette smoking, diabetes mellitus, heart disease).

• Positive history of blunt trauma to the perineal region, such as bicycle riding or pelvic fracture.

• Erectile dysfunction due to pure cavernosal arterial insufficiency, this is, failure of the erection chambers to fill with blood.

• Erectile dysfunction *not* related to psychological, hormonal, neurologic (i.e., failure to initiate an erection) or corporalveno-occlusive dysfunction (venous leak).

• Presence of arterial abnormalities in the cavernosal arteries as determined by appropriate imaging studies.

A problem as significant as arterial insufficiency (i.e., inadequate blood flow to the penis) is the leakage of blood out of the penis, thus preventing the penis from becoming engorged and erect. The surgical procedure to correct this problem is called *venous ligation*, which cuts off some of the veins that carry blood out of the penis and thereby puts the vascular system in balance. Cancer survivors indicate that this does not work very well or for very long. These procedures work only when erectile dysfunction results from simple vascular injury. They are usually not options for prostate cancer patients who have had surgery or radiation.

One report was that, although initial recovery within six months after surgery, "the long-term success rate of penile vein ligation is only about 20 percent."

A new process has evolved that was first used in 2000 called *venous embolization*. Generally, a vein is blocked by clotting or being radiologically cauterized in the penis. A similar technique has been used highly successfully in women where the uterine fibroids are starved of nutrients by stopping the blood supply to them. A 2001 European trial showed that twenty-six percent of men had a good response at about two years. When patients had additional therapy, such as orals or injections, the success rate rose to forty-four percent. Since men in the test were selected based on maintenance flow, intracavernous oxygen, and other factors, the technique may be effective only in a select group.

New target areas for erectile dysfunction research

The information presented here is rather technical in nature. It is included to provide an indication of the diversity of approaches being pursued to develop new treatments for erectile dysfunction.

The research discussed in this section may offer hope to men for whom current therapies are not ideal or do not work. There are at least seven areas of research, some of which are extremely broad and from which several different products may become available, and others which are focused on one type of receptor to cause erections, much in the same manner as PDE-5 inhibitors do now. Many of the medications being produced through this research will enter clinical research before the year 2010. (The FDA process for approving new medications is long in order to assure that the user will not be harmed.)

New directions for means of helping men obtain erections seem to focus on chemicals that make the central nervous system cause actions in muscles in the genital organs.

Oral therapies may act:

- *Centrally* (in the brain) to stimulate receptors that regulate sexual functions.
- *Peripherally* (at the specific site in the body where an action is desired, in this case, the penis).
- *Both centrally and peripherally.*

In 1998, apomorphine was being developed as a sublingual (under the tongue) drug that would work on the central nervous system. Although available in Europe, the FDA rejected it twice for use in the United States. A recent paper noted that apomorphine sublingual is most effective in men with short-term ED who still have some erectile function. One company, Nastech Pharmaceutical Co., Inc. is developing an intranasal apomorphine. The nasal approach is being pursued because it targets the release of oxytocin that ultimately causes relaxation of the penile muscle (required for the penis to become engorged) and the flow of blood. Two other companies are doing clinical investigations into second-generation dopamine agonists. Pharmacia is working on "sumanirole" and the Abbott research effort is ABT 724.

At this point, several other pharmaceutical companies are known to be working on other compounds that will act on the central nervous system to deal with ED. Compounds that may become future treatments include melanocortin (PT-141, Palatin, previously discussed under new products in development, is one of them). Studies have shown that PT-141 will cause erections even when the man is not aroused. However, with arousal the percentage of men achieving erections increased to two-thirds in a clinical trial. Other drug therapies are targeting growth hormone–releasing peptide receptors, and drugs that would be aimed at 5-hydroxyltryptamine receptors.

In the area of central and peripheral agents are alpha adrenergic blockers, which would continue the release of the chemical that maintains the erection. Vasomax (Zonagen) might have been an early competitor to the other orals but, as previously mentioned, development has been suspended. Under the label Invicorp™, Senetek PLC is combining a vasoactive intestinal polypeptide and phentolamine as an injectable medication. Two other developments in this class of compounds being developed are delequamine and atipamezole.

One company is developing a compound, NMI 870, which combines the alpha-blocker yohimbine with L-arginine. L-arginine is a precursor for nitric oxide, which is needed for erections. Although medical thinking is that one cannot take L-arginine alone to obtain erections, it may enhance the effect of yohimbine.

Peripheral activation of erections has been primarily achieved with intracavernosal injections. However, two companies are researching compounds that will inhibit Rho-kinase, which keeps the penis flaccid. In one clinical trial patients taking both the rho-kinase inhibitor and sildenafil (Viagra®) had erections that lasted almost twenty-three minutes compared to about nine minutes for the inhibitor alone and almost ten minutes for the placebo. Other research concerns yet another chemical that is responsible for activating nitric oxide, the enzyme-soluble guanyl cyclase.

Another research route is evidenced by Eli Lilly's research in developing pinacidil. The compound is a selective potassium channel activator that could be administered both orally and by injection. This compound would address another route for obtaining relaxation of penile smooth muscle, thus permitting increased blood flow and subsequently an erection.

Nonapproved and Off Label Treatments

9

Key Points

✔ *Use of drugs, or of drugs and devices in combination, may provide more effective treatment of erectile dysfunction for some men.*

✔ *Combining therapies should be undertaken only when prescribed by a physician, and the doctor's directions must be carefully followed because there is more than one set of side effects.*

✔ *Do not take medications for an off label use unless prescribed by your doctor for such use.*

✔ *While herbal products are natural, they are not necessarily harmless. If you wish to try an herbal remedy or supplement, educate yourself about the product, and discuss it with your doctor before you start taking it.*

✔ *Herbal products are not FDA-regulated. Consumers cannot be sure of the contents, the amounts of each substance in a product, or the side effects.*

The treatment landscape for erectile dysfunction gets more crowded each day as new therapies become available. Even so, the growing number of treatments do not solve every man's problem. Every treatment seems to work well for some men, partially for others, and not at all for still others. In addition, even though a medication may have the desired result, the side effects may force the patient and doctor to stop using it and look for alternatives.

As with treatments for many other diseases or conditions, doctors have begun to create combinations of therapies sometimes referred to as *ED cocktails*. Drug combinations are generally not approved as combination therapies by the U.S. Food and Drug Administration (FDA). Although some of the medications used in these combinations were developed for the purpose of treating ED, they were developed to be used only as a single agent, not in combination. Other medications were developed to treat one illness or condition and then were found to have the side effect of improving erectile function. These medications are not approved by the FDA for treating ED, at least at the outset, although over time the agency's approval may be obtained if the manufacturer conducts the appropriate studies. Use of a medication for a purpose for which it is not approved is legal when the medication is prescribed by a doctor; such uses are known as *off label* use, because they are outside the approved uses described on the medication's label.

This chapter describes the spectrum of medications and supplements that are not approved by the FDA for treatment of erectile dysfunction, as well as combinations of medications and/or devices that patients use, some of which are approved and some not. It is important that men and their partners be presented with all available information so that they do not rely solely on anecdotal information that may be incomplete or incorrect. This material is for information only, and before using a nonapproved medication or device, or medications/devices in combination, a man should always discuss the potential positive and negative effects with a qualified medical professional.

Combination Therapies

Combination therapies using sildenafil (Viagra®)

At the time these studies were done, sildenafil (Viagra®) was the only PDE-5 inhibitor approved for use. Since then vardenafil (Levitra®) and tadalafil (Cialis®) have become available. If you wish to try a combination therapy with any of these drugs, consult with your doctor.

Sildenafil (Viagra®) and doxazosin (Cardura). Almost eighty percent of patients with nonorganic erectile dysfunction showed significant improvement with this combination therapy.

Doxazosin is an antihypertensive medication and can cause significant reduction in blood pressure. Doxazosin is an alpha-adrenergic blocker. Besides lowering blood pressure, it relaxes the muscles in the prostate and bladder neck, making it easier to urinate.

The risk of stroke and heart attack is highest in the morning when the blood pressure is highest. By taking antihypertensive medication in the evening, it reaches maximum effect when the body most needs it to keep the blood pressure under control. Cardura works over a twenty-four-hour period, and loses some of its effectiveness toward the end of the period.

Viagra® lowers blood pressure over a four-hour period. Since each of these medications drops the blood pressure, the key problem is that the combination of the two could drop pressure levels dangerously low, causing heart problems.

Your urologist and internist can jointly resolve the problem. Taking Viagra® for nocturnal erections to avoid penile muscle atrophy may be part of a penile rehabilitation protocol (see Chapter 8, page 147). Alternatives are using injections or a vacuum device to provide penile rehabilitation.

Sildenafil (Viagra®) and apomorphine (Ixense and Uprima, in Europe, Latin America, and Asia only). This combination therapy is used to combine a centrally acting dopamine-agonist medication (apomorphine) with a peripherally acting agent (sildenafil) when neither one works well or at all separately. The probability of an erection increases because, while Viagra® blocks enzymes resulting in relaxation of the smooth muscles in the corpus cavernosum, apomorphine works through receptors in the brain to enhance the body's responsiveness to erectogenic stimuli.

Sildenafil (Viagra®) and a tension ring. Some men have found that although Viagra® helps them obtain an erection, they are not able to maintain it. In all likelihood, the problem is venous leakage because blood flow is either insufficient to compress the veins or the penis has lost some elasticity. In much the same way that MUSE® and Actis® evolved as a combination, doctors prescribe a tension ring like those used with vacuum systems or MUSE® to enable men to retain their erection after taking Viagra®.

We can assume that doctors may prescribe tension rings for Levitra® and Cialis® patients who cannot maintain their erections. Use of a constriction ring is a short-term solution during a sexual episode, usually less than thirty minutes, for retaining the erection. Other side effects are noted in the "Devices" section in Chapter 8 (page 147).

Sildenafil (Viagra®) and a vacuum erection device. Patients have used Viagra® in conjunction with a vacuum erection device (VED) when a VED alone was unsatisfactory. In this instance, one possibility is that the Viagra® was needed to relax the cavernosal muscles so that the corpora cavernosa could become more fully engorged.

Sildenafil (Viagra®) and intraurethral prostaglandin E-1 (MUSE®). Generally, men are reluctant to use injection therapy for ED. For this reason, researchers carried out a study reported in a 2002 paper in the *International Journal of Impotence Research*. They carried out this combination therapy for thirty months with twenty-eight patients, none of whom had successful erections with either Viagra® or MUSE® alone. "After initiating a combination therapy, at 30 months, all 28 patients were reporting erections sufficient for vaginal penetration, with 3.6 intercourse episodes per month." The researchers concluded that "combination therapy with MUSE® and sildenafil (Viagra®) may be more efficacious" for patients who do not want injections and where single treatments fail.

Sildenafil (Viagra®) and intracavernosal injection (Caverject®). Some men have tried Viagra®/Caverject® combinations and found the erections last longer than using either of the two alone. The oral medication is taken and followed by the intercavernosal injection about a half-hour later. The injection provides an erection without arousal; however, subsequent arousal seems to enhance the erection. In one case, the man subsequently used Levitra® in place of Viagra®. He found that the erection lasts longer with Levitra® and there are fewer side effects.

Combination therapies using yohimbine hydrochloride

The following two combinations are discussed because many practitioners continue to prescribe yohimbine, even though many studies have concluded that it is no better than a placebo. For more information see the yohimbine discussion under oral medications in Chapter 8 (page 123).

Yohimbine and L-arginine glutamate. L-arginine alone, according to Dr. J. Douglas Trapp, President of Impotence Consultants Inc., does not work and he doubts that one could take the high dosage required for it to have any effect. However, a "double-blind, placebo-controlled, three-way crossover, randomized clinical trial" compared the efficacy and safety of the L-arginine-yohimbine combination with that of yohimbine alone and a placebo. The researchers concluded "that the on-demand oral administration of the 6 g L-arginine glutamate and 6 mg yohimbine combination is effective in improving erectile function in patients with *mild to moderate* [emphasis added] ED. It appears to be a promising addition to first-line therapy for ED."

Yohimbine and naltrexone. In 2002, the National Institutes of Health initiated a study "to evaluate the effects and safety of a potential novel treatment combination for ED consisting of both, ... yohimbine ... and naltrexone." Naltrexone is extensively used to counter addiction.

Study participants will be normal, healthy men up to fifty years of age, indicating that the initial results may not apply to the majority of men treated for prostate cancer. However, the researchers expect that the study could be applied also to patients with ED of different causes (e.g., organic, psychogenic and others).

Off Label Drug Usage

In the course of using some drugs, side effects are noted that may help alleviate or treat another condition. The following medications are reported to have promise in dealing with some aspects of erectile dysfunction. These medications are neither recognized nor approved for treating the "side effect" applications. Nevertheless, they are noted here because physicians are discussing their use in treating ED. It is legal for a doctor to prescribe a medication for off label use.

Dopamine receptor agonists

Dostinex and others are the subject of emails being circulated that say they increase sexual desire and improve a man's ability to have multiple orgasms. Three medications in this group are used to reduce prolactin levels. This treatment is especially appropriate for men whose prolactin level is high, because of pituitary malfunction, or who are taking medications that can compromise pituitary function. These include drugs for psychological problems, hypertension, and even stomach disorders. By lowering the prolactin level, to get it in the normal range, the testosterone level increases and so does sexual desire.

The three available medications are bromocriptine (Parlodel), pergolide (Permax), and cabergoline (Dostinex). Of the three, Dostinex has been most often touted as giving men sexual stamina for multiple orgasms. Dr. Charles Myers noted (in the *Prostate Forum*, Vol. 6, No. 12) that the drug cabergoline (Dostinex) was very useful in reducing cancer cell growth by blocking the production of prolactin by the brain. One of the "good" side effects is that it increases libido. However, it can cause mild diarrhea at the onset of use. Dosage for its labeled use is small and only twice a week.

As yet there have been no clinical trials to show that these drugs have the claimed effects or that, even if they do have the promoted sexual effects, they are applicable to men who have been treated for prostate cancer.

Herbal Products and Dietary Supplements

Herbal supplements fit the category of home remedies that many people utilize. They are used widely to deal with a broad variety of medical conditions and just for feeling good.

Herbal products are sometimes referred to as *complementary* or *alternative medicine* (CAM). Less well-known is the term *integrative medicine*. According to the National Institutes of Health (NIH), National Center for Complementary and Alternative Medicine, the definitions are:

• Complementary medicine comprises therapies used together with conventional medicine.

• Alternative medicine consists of therapies used in place of conventional medicine.

• Integrative medicine combines mainstream medical therapies and CAM therapies for which there is some high-quality scientific evidence of safety and effectiveness.

However, a cautionary note must be added before discussing herbal supplements that may contribute to alleviating some degree of ED. Every so often, there is another instance of dietary supplements causing untoward side effects, even death, or exploiting a group such as sports figures with promises of performance enhancement. The danger may lie in the promoted substance or in undeclared substances included in the pill, capsule, or liquid. Another possibility is that what you buy won't hurt you but you may not get the results you are paying for.

In the June 2003 issue of *Prostate Cancer Communication*, Mark Moyad addressed the question of " ... which dietary supplements (if any) may help men with ED?" He begins his article with the issue of quality control, noting "Currently supplements sold in the U.S. are not subject to specific standards or quality control testing." "Therefore, without any adequate independent and universal randomized quality control studies ..." the quality and the quantity of active ingredients of any dietary supplement are unknown. Other countries, especially Germany, actually treat supplements more like prescription drugs. Supplements are usually taken on a patient's initiative, and, given there is no regulation of dietary supplements, consumers must be aware of what and why they are buying the product, and should purchase products only from established manufacturers and reputable outlets.

Several herbal products are reputed to, and *may* actually, help loving. Our comments are not meant to be comprehensive. Literature, emails, and anecdotes abound concerning products that are libido lifters, that will give you King Kong–type erections, and that will drive your partner wild with excitement. We don't know anything about these products and suspect that most of the related information is marketing hype.

We will tell you about some products that have been discussed in the prostate cancer literature. We are not recommending that you take any product. While herbal products are natural, they are not always harmless. They may worsen a current condition, have bad side effects, or interfere with medications you are taking.

In general, if you use herbal products, you should buy the standardized extract of the herb made by a reputable company. Several studies have reported that some companies' labels are misleading. Products made by reputable companies will be reliably labeled.

Readers interested in more information on herbs and supplements should consult *The American Pharmaceutical Association Practical Guide to Natural Medicines* by Andrea Peirce, which covers more than three hundred herbs and some supplements. The book provides the scientific and common names for each herb, the ailment(s) it's recommended for, the forms in which it is available, the commonly prescribed dosages, and information on the herb's effectiveness and safety based on scientific study.

Ginkgo

Studies have shown that ginkgo may have therapeutic effects. Ginkgolide B was isolated by Harvard scientists in the 1980s. Ginkgo's effect is to dramatically increase blood flow to the brain, and it is purportedly able to improve "blood flow through peripheral arteries lined with plaque."

One 1998 article stated that because it increases blood flow and circulation, ginkgo may work in a way similar to Viagra®. *Psychology Today*, in its October 1998 issue, reported: "In one recent study, 50 patients with impotence were given ginkgo, and after six months, an astonishing one-half had regained sexual vigor. ... [M]en taking ginkgo need to be patient, since significant results may not show up for several months. It takes time for the body to repair damaged blood vessels ... ."

Anecdotal confirmation comes from several people who responded to our article in the January–February 1998 issue of the Education Center for Prostate Cancer Patients (ECPCP) newsletter, saying that doubling the normal dose of ginkgo (from sixty to one hundred twenty milligrams twice a day) enabled them to obtain erections. Ginkgo is manufactured by many herbal product companies and is widely available even in supermarkets. As noted above, consumers should buy products from reputable manufacturers and in established outlets. A 2000 test of fourteen samples by the World Health Organization (WHO) "showed that in 11 cases, the products did not contain all the active ingredients associated with *Ginkgo biloba* leaf extract as specified in standards set by the WHO ... ." Only one of the samples had the recommended level of active ingredients. Prospective consumers are advised to read the labels carefully and research any brand they are interested in buying.

L-arginine

L-arginine is noted above as being included in a study in combination with yohimbine. However, in one study, forty percent of the patients taking twenty-eight hundred milligrams per day for two weeks said they had improved erections. But the patients were young and had good vascular function. In a second trial, patients who took fifteen hundred milligrams daily for two weeks did not notice any improvement. In the third trial, thirty-one percent of the patients said their erections improved after taking five grams daily for six weeks. Statistically, the difference is significant. Except for some patients experiencing a drop in their blood pressure, no other side effects were noticed.

Kava

The kava plant has been widely reported to be a natural relaxant that does not dull the mind, as many such substances do. As a result, kava seems to permit an individual's natural sexual appetite to surface. Supplements containing the herbal ingredient kava are promoted for relaxation (e.g., to relieve stress, anxiety, and tension, sleeplessness, menopausal symptoms, and other conditions.)

However, kava-containing products have been associated with liver-related injuries, including hepatitis, cirrhosis, and liver failure. In March 2002, the FDA Center for Food Safety and Applied Nutrition (CFSAN) notified healthcare professionals and consumers of the potential risk of severe liver injury associated with the use of kava-containing dietary supplements. The warning said that persons who have liver disease or liver problems, or persons who are taking drug products that can affect the liver, should consult a physician before using kava-containing supplements. Liver-associated risks have prompted regulatory agencies in other countries, including those in Germany, Switzerland, France, Canada, and the United Kingdom, to take action ranging from warning consumers about the potential risks of kava use to removing kava-containing products from the marketplace. Although liver damage appears to be rare, FDA believes consumers should be informed of this potential risk.

In addition to physical issues, one of the biggest problems for both prostate cancer survivors and others is that psychological factors limit a man's capability for intercourse. Chemicals in the kava plant are said to ease anxiety and relax muscles. Concurrently, erections are facilitated when the psychological barrier is lessened, because there is less anxiety about getting an erection. Rather than risking liver damage or the other side effects of kava, men who might experience anxiety in lovemaking should consult their physician for other options to reduce anxiety.

Korean Red Ginseng

A Korean study investigated the efficacy of Korean red ginseng on forty-five patients who had erectile dysfunction. Working on a standard clinical trial protocol, they found that the men who were on the ginseng did much better, specifically regarding penetration and maintaining the erection. The fact that penetration had improved could suggest that blood flow was better for a high level of rigidity. Generally, maintaining the erection is accomplished by controlling venous outflow. The study concluded that "Korean red ginseng can be as [sic] effective alternative for treating male erectile dysfunction." Although the patients had ED, it is not known whether they were representative in any respect of patients that have been treated for prostate cancer.

Putting It All Together

All beginnings are hard. If you have trouble figuring out how to get started, maybe the examples of the following couples will give you ideas. As always, you have to adjust the strategy to the participants, so it depends on what kind of a relationship you and your partner have, and what your personalities are.

We'll introduce you to three couples.

Romeo and Juliet

The first couple had been married for twenty-six years and had always been very romantic. Loving was very important to both partners. We'll call them Romeo and Juliet, although they are a bit older than Shakespeare's lovers.

Before Romeo had surgery, he and Juliet talked about the fact that, no matter what damage the surgery caused to his potency, they would find a way to make love afterward. So they both knew the other was interested.

After surgery, Romeo lost most of his erectile capability. They decided to use this as an opportunity to rediscover each other. They agreed that they both would learn together and try new things, knowing that some things would work and some wouldn't. They started over, as if they were new lovers, getting to know each other's bodies all over again.

They consciously slowed down the pace of their lovemaking and found that it became a completely different experience—one they liked very much! They began to read passages from books to each other, which at least one of them found erotic. They got some good laughs when they discovered that they didn't always agree on what was erotic—but most of the time they did. They also tried shots and Viagra®, and they are planning to try Levitra® and Cialis®; they continue to use them, but only on "special occasions." They're using more variety in their sex life, making love with oral sex, manual stimulation, and lots of sensual touching. The results? Juliet says:

> I used to get frustrated sometimes because Romeo was so goal-oriented. I always wanted much more touching and sensuality. Most people would shake their heads in disbelief if I told them that now I've got everything I wanted—but it's true! I enjoy lovemaking much more now and really feel that Romeo has become an even better lover than before. We've always had a good and healthy relationship, but now I feel that our relationship is even deeper. And lovemaking is even more important to us now than it had been in the last few years.

Romeo echoes her feelings:

> I was not happy when I realized that this capability that I used to think of as an essential part of me was drastically reduced. Not making love was never an option for us—whatever it took, we would do it together. But I thought that she would get most of the pleasure, and it would be mostly frustration and disappointment for me. It really hasn't happened that way. We make better love today than we ever have. I've learned things about my body and hers that I wish I'd known thirty years ago. We've found some pretty nifty places and ways to touch each other that send us both into orbit. Don't get me wrong: There are times when we both really miss the old no-fuss erections. So sometimes we use Caverject or Viagra®, but that's a special treat. And most of the time we're very happy with our unaided lovemaking. With the aids, you just tend to do the same two or three things. Without them, you let your imagination take you wherever it will. It's amazing how many different things you'll come up with."

Napoleon and Josephine

Our second couple had a very traditional relationship and rather conservative sexual habits. Since he's a military man, we'll call him Napoleon and her Josephine. Napoleon was devastated when he realized his potency was affected. He withdrew and didn't even mention sex for eight months. Josephine went on a slow but steady campaign to show her love and support and to rebuild his confidence, but it took quite a while.

While giving Napoleon a massage because he seemed "so tense," Josephine found that he was okay with (nonsexual) touching. She finally figured out how to talk to him about this topic: She played on his military background.

She presented the enemy: absence of lovemaking due to impotence. His key ally: Josephine. His strengths: coming up with a strategy and a battle plan, and executing it with persistence. Their challenge: Napoleon's treatment had been like an earthquake to his body. It had changed the terrain. The first step was to explore the terrain. Josephine is a very creative and convincing lady, and Napoleon bought into the idea of the plan. It included, of course, a communication plan (you must always talk to each other) and a contract (absolutely no putting down the partner if something they tried did not work). There would be heavy penalties if the contract was broken: If she broke it, she'd have to attend a hockey game with him, and if he broke it, he'd have to accompany her to the mall while she shopped for clothes.

They started with a session exploring the unknown terrain of his body. His sensitive spots had definitely shifted. He was surprised to find that he was very aroused by being touched in some places far from the genital area. He kept looking for the erection, and Josephine kept telling him not to worry about it, but just to enjoy the touching. Their third touch session was spontaneous and involved touching by both partners.

Josephine also gave him more hugs and other spontaneous demonstrations of affection. She tried to wear clothes that appealed to him. Slowly, she "warmed him up" to the idea of lovemaking in a new way. She made sure he understood what made her feel good and guided him to the appropriate places, told him how to touch her for the greatest pleasure. They tried things they had never done before: oral sex, manual stimulation, vibrators, lubricants, and other things they didn't want to tell us in detail. And they always kept touching.

When Viagra® came out, Napoleon tried it, but he got bad headaches. His doctor recommended shots, and Napoleon now takes tri-mix about once a month. The rest of the time he and Josephine engage in their newfound variety of lovemaking. They dress up a little for each other and make occasional "dates" with each other.

Napoleon comments, "It's almost embarrassing to think that we're in our sixties trying all these new things, but it has really recharged our batteries. In some ways we're like newlyweds now. I never knew I had such a sexy wife." Josephine says, "I have really great orgasms, and I'm not shy about showing him. It's important that he knows how much pleasure he gives me." But what's most important to her is that she was able to break through the barrier that had been created by Napoleon's pain over the erectile dysfunction.

Bill and Jill

Let's call our third couple Bill and Jill. Bill had a combination of hormone treatment, vaccination, and radiation. His hormone treatment was stopped as soon as possible because of the terrible side effects he was experiencing—not just low libido, but feeling depressed within a certain time period after each hormone shot. Even after stopping the hormone treatment, he still felt extremely tired and weak.

Being a positive, can-do person, he decided to counteract the fatigue by exercising. Using a treadmill was rather boring, and, after he'd watched every video they had while exercising, Jill came up with the idea that she would read to him while he was exercising. One of the books she read to him described the sensual sex approach. They had relied on Viagra® since Bill's treatment and decided to try without it. The first time they tried "sensual sex" was such an intense experience that they both cried.

Bill says, "It was an awakening for me realizing that intercourse was not the only way, or the most important way, to have a sexual relationship. And that we could both get such physical and emotional satisfaction and enjoyment from being with each other." Erection and intercourse are much less of a concern now, replaced by the focus on intimacy, sharing, sexual touching, and "erection-free orgasms." It has opened up a new dimension of their sexual and emotional intimacy, and enabled them to grow further as a couple, taking their relationship to a new level.

These couples show that, if you're interested in rebuilding your physical relationship, you can do it. The key ingredients are an understanding of your partner, the understanding of each other's bodies and likes and dislikes, creativity, and the willingness to try new things. A lot of touching and slowing down the pace of love-making also help most couples.

Love and caring for each other, a sense of romance and adventure, and making love in a way that involves your body, mind, and soul, and all your senses can revive the sizzle in your relationship. Treat each other as the sexual beings you are, and enjoy it!

We wish that each one of you will achieve the potential that you have. Cervantes wrote, "If only dreams and reality weren't so far apart." We submit that when you want good loving, you can realize your dream.

We wish you a happy, healthy, sensual, and loving relationship!

—Barbara and Ralph Alterowitz

Appendix A:
Treatments for Erectile
Dysfunction

Table A-1. Medications

Brand Name	Generic Name	Route of Administration	Mode of Action	Manufacturer	Availability	See Page No.
Alprox-TD®	alprostadil (synthetic prostaglandin E-1 [PGE1])	Topical	Vasodilator	NexMed	Asia (trade name Befar)	129
Bi-mix, Trimix	papaverine + phentolamine, papaverine + phentolamine + PGE1	Intracavernosal injection	Vasodilator	Special formulations	United States	143
Quad-mix	papaverine + phentolamine PGE1 + forskolin					
Caverject®	alprostadil (PGE-1)	Intracavernosal injection	Vasodilator	Pfizer	United States, Europe	139
Cialis	tadalafil	Oral	PDE-5 inhibitor	Lilly	Europe	117
EDEX	alprostadil (PGE-1)	Intracavernosal injection	Vasodilator	Schwarz Pharma	United States, Europe	140
Invicorp	phentolamine + vasoactive intestinal peptide+	Intracavernosal injection	Vasodilator	Senetek	United Kingdom, Denmark?	142
Levitra	vardenafil	Oral	PDE-5 inhibitor	Bayer / Glaxo	United States, Europe	115
MUSE®	alprostadil (PGE-1)	Intraurethral	Vasodilator	Vivus	United States, Europe	132
Topiglan®	alprostadil (PGE-1)	Topical	Vasodilator	MachroChem	Phase III trials in United States	128
Uprima, Ixense	apomorphine	Oral	Dopamine receptor agonist	TAP Pharmaceutical Products, Inc.	Europe, Asia	125
Vasomax	phentolamine	Oral	Nonselective adrenergic receptor blockade	Zonagen	Trials suspended in United States	126
Viagra	sildenafil	Oral	PDE-5 inhibitor	Pfizer	United States, Europe	120
Yohimbine (various brand names)	yohimbine	Oral	alpha adrenergic receptor antagonist	Numerous manufacturers	Generally available under different trade names, such as: Actibine, Aphrodyne, Reveryvl, Reverzine, Yobine, Yocon	123

190

Table A-2. Devices

Brand Name	Generic Name	Route of Administration	Mode of Action	Manufacturer	Availability	See Page No.
AMS Ambicor® AMS 700CX™/CXR™ AMS 700 Ultrex/Ultrex	Penile implant	Surgery	Inflatable	American Medical Systems	United States	160
Malleable \ 600M/650 DURA II	Penile Implant	Surgery	Malleable	American Medical Systems	United States	160
Rejoyn	Support sleeve	External	External support of	American Medical	United States	147
Touch® II; Response™ II Vitality™/Vitality™ Plus Assist™	Vacuum erection device [VED]	External	Vacuum (negative pressure)	Augusta Medical Systems	United States	151
Vacurect™ Rx Vacurect™ OTC	Vacuum erection device [VED]	External	Vacuum (negative pressure)	Vacurect Manufacturing (Pty) Ltd., distributed by Bonro Medical in United States	United States	157
ImpoAid™VTU-1 ImpoAid™VTU-E ImpoAid™Deluxe	Vacuum erection device [VED]	External	Vacuum (negative pressure)	Encore Medical Products	United States	153
Acu-Form®	Penile implant	Surgery	Malleable	Mentor	United States	161
Titan™; Alpha I®	Penile implant	Surgery	Inflatable	Mentor	United States	161
VED Ultra® VED Classic®	Vacuum erection device [VED]	External	Vacuum (negative pressure)	Mission Pharmacal	United States	154
ErecAid Esteem™	Vacuum erection device [VED]	External	Vacuum (negative pressure)	Endocare	United States	156
Rejoyn; MVP-700 IVP-600 Bos 2000-2	Vacuum erection device [VED]	External	Vacuum (negative pressure)	Pos-T-Vac	United States	155
Actis®	Constriction band	External	Adjustable constriction band	Vivuc	United States	133, 140

191

Table A-3. Combination Therapies

	Drug Combination	Mode of Action	See Page No.
Combinations with sildenafil*	Sildenafil + Actis®	PDE-5 inhibitor + constriction	176
	Sildenafil + MUSE®	PDE-5 inhibitor + vasodilator	176
	Sildenafil + apomorphine	PDE-5 inhibitor + CNS stimulant	175
	Sildenafil + Doxazosin	PDE-5 inhibitor + alpha 1 blocker (vasodilator)	175
	Sildenafil + vacuum device	PDE-5 inhibitor + pump	176
	Sildenafil + alprostadil injection	PDE-5 inhibitor + vasodilator	176
Combinations with yohimbine	Yohimbine + naltrexone	Vasodilator + opiate receptor blocker	177
	Yohimbine + 1-arginine	Vasodilator + nitric oxide precursor	177
Other combinations	Apomorphine + alpha adrenoceptor antagonists (phentolamine)	CNS stimulant + nonselective alpha adrenergic blocker (vasodilator)	NA in U.S.

*When these combinations were first reported, sildenafil was the only PDE-5 inhibitor available. Some doctors may use other drugs of this type that have recently become available.

Table A-4. Non-FDA-Approved Therapies

Brand Name	Generic Name	Route of Administration	Mode of Action	Manufacturer	See Page No.
Dostinex	cabergoline	Oral	Dopamine receptor agonist	Pfizer (Pharmacia)	178
Desyrel	trazodone	Oral	Serotonin uptake inhibitor	Bristol Myers Squibb	193

These drugs should only be used for erectile dysfunction if prescribed by your own physician for that purpose.
These drugs are not labeled for use as erectile dysfunction treatments.

Table A-5. New Medications in Development

Brand Name	Generic Name	Route of Administration	Mode of Action	Manufacturer	See Page No.
GPI 1485	Neuroimmunophilin ligand	n/a	Neuroregenerative activity	Guilford Pharmaceuticals	145
PT-141	Melanocortin	Intranasal	Central nervous system stimulation	Palatin Technologies	146
	Oxytocin & Oxytocin receptors	n/a	Central Nervous System stimulation of specific receptors		146, 170
	Growth hormone releasing peptide receptors	n/a	Central Nervous System stimulation of specific receptors		146, 170
	5-hydroxytryptamine receptors	n/a	Inhibition of serotinin uptake by specific receptors		146, 170
	Guanylyl cyclase	n/a	Enzyme in penile tissue		146, 170
	Rho-kinase	n/a	Enzyme in penile tissue		146, 170
	Human arginase II	n/a	Enzyme in penile tissue		146, 170

*n/a = information not available

Appendix B:
Manufacturers of Erectile Dysfunction Products

American Medical Systems
Penile prostheses
Brand Names: AMS 700CX™/CXR™; 700 Ultrex; Ambicor®;
Malleable 600M™/650M™, DURA II™
    10700 Bren Road West
    Minnetonka, MN 55343
    800-328-3881
    952-933-4666
    www.visitams.com

American MedTech
Penile support sleeve
Tension rings
Brand Name: Rejoyn (both products)
    5217 Wayzata Boulevard #140
    St. Louis Park, MN 55416
    612-543-5630
    www.rejoyn.com

Augusta Medical Systems
Vacuum therapy systems
Brand Name: Touch II®; Response II®, Vitality™/Vitality™ Plus,
Assist™
    1027 Broad Street
    Augusta, GA 30903
    800-827-8382
    www.augustams.com

Bayer
Oral medication
Brand Name: Levitra®
400 Morgan Lane
West Haven, CT 06516
800-468-0894
www.bayer.com, www.levitra.com

Bonro Medical, Inc. (Distributor for Vacurect Manufacturing [Pty] Ltd.)
Brand Names: Vacurect™ Rx, Vacurect™ OTC
P.O. Box 211610
Martinez, GA 30917
866-692-6676, 877-266-7699
www.bonro.com

Encore Medical Products
Vacuum therapy system
Brand Names: ImpoAid™ VTU-1, ImpoAid™ VTU-E, ImpoAid™ Deluxe
9900 Corporate Campus Drive, Suite 3000
Louisville, KY 40223
877-853-5717
www.impoaid.com

Lilly
Oral medication
Brand Name: Cialis®
22021 20th Avenue SE
Bothell, WA 98021
206-485-1900
www.cialis.com

MacroChem
Topical
Brand Name: Topiglan®
110 Hartwell Avenue, Suite 2
Lexington, MA 02421-3134
781-862-4003
www.macrochem.com

Mentor Corp.
Penile prostheses
Brand Names: Alpha I® Inflatable Penile Prosthesis; Titan™ Inflatable Penile Prothesis; Excel™ Inflatable Penile Prosthesis; Mark II® Inflatable Penile Prosthesis; Acu-Form® Penile Prosthesis; Malleable Penile Prothesis
201 Mentor Drive
Santa Barbara, CA 93111
805-525-0245
www.mentorcorp.com, www.straighttalk.mentorcorp.com

Mission Pharmacal
Vacuum therapy system
Brand Names: VED Ultra®, VED Classic®
10999 Interstate Highway 10 West
San Antonio, TX 78230
800-531-3333
www.missionpharmacal.com

NexMed
Topical
Brand Name: Alprox-TD®
350 Corporate Boulevard
Robbinsville, NJ 08691
609-208-9688
www.nexmed.com

Palatin Technologies, Inc.
Intranasal (product in development)
Brand Name: n/a
4C Cedar Brook Drive
Cranbury, NJ 08512
609-495-2200
www.palatin.com

Pfizer
Oral medication
Brand Name: Viagra®
235 East 42nd Street
New York, NY 10017
888-4VIAGRA, 888-733-2009
www.viagra.com

Pfizer (formerly Pharmacia-Upjohn)
Intracavernosal injection
Brand Name: Caverject®
100 Route 206 North
Peapack, NJ 07977
888-691-6813
800-879-3477
www.caverject.com

Pos-T-Vac
Vacuum erection device
Brand Names: Pos-T-Vac™ IVP-600, Pos-T-Vac MVP-700™,
Rejoyn, Bos 2000-2
1701 North 14th Avenue—P.O. Box 1436
Dodge City, KS 67801
800-279-7434
www.postvac.com

Schwarz Pharma
Intracavernosal injection
Brand Name: EDEX®
6140 W. Executive Drive
Mequon, WI 53092
800-558-5114
www.schwarzusa.com

Senetek
Intracavernosal injection
Brand Name: Invicorp™
620 Airpark Road
Napa, CA 94558
707-226-3900
www.senetekplc.com

TAP Pharmaceutical Products, Inc.
Oral medication
Brand Name: Uprima®, Ixense
675 North Field Drive
Lake Forest, IL 60045
800-621-1020
www.tap.com

TIMM (a subsidiary of Endocare)
Vacuum therapy system
Brand Name: ErecAid™ Esteem™
6585 City West Parkway
Eden Prairie, MN 55344
800-438-8592
www.timmmedical.com

Vivus, Inc.
Intraurethral suppository
Brand Name: MUSE®
Adjustable constriction loop
Brand Name: Actis®
1172 Castro Street
Mountain View, CA 94040
888-367-6873
650-934-5200
www.vivus.com

Zonagen
Oral medication
Brand Name: Vasomax
2408 Timeberloch Place
The Woodlands, TX 77380
281-367-5892
www.zonagen.com

Appendix C:
Resources

Here are sources of information on sexual health and prostate disease. This is by no means a complete listing and is provided only as a starting point. Many Internet sites listed here have links to other relevant sites.

American Association for Marriage and Family Therapy (AAMFT)
112 S Alfred Street
Alexandria, VA 22314-3061
703-838-9808
www.aamft.org

American Association of Sex Educators, Counselors, and Therapists (AASECT)
P.O. Box 5488
Richmond, VA 23220-0488
www.aasect.org

American Foundation for Urologic Disease (AFUD)
Sexual Function Health Council
1000 Corporate Boulevard, Suite 410
Linthicum, MD 21090
800-828-7866
410-689-39907
www.impotence.org
www.afud.org
www.prostatehealth.com

American Urological Association (AUA)
1120 N Charles Street
Baltimore, MD 21201-5559
410-727-1100
www.auanet.org
www.urologyhealth.org (patient information Web site)

Education Center for Prostate Cancer Patients (ECPCP)
380 N. Broadway, Suite 304
Jericho, NY 11753
516-942-5000
www.ecpcp.org

**National Cancer Institute (part of the National
Institutes of Health [NIH])**
NCI Public Inquiries Office
6116 Executive Boulevard, MSC8322, Suite 3036A
Bethesda, MD 20892-8322
www.cancer.gov

The National Women's Health Resource Center
157 Broad Street, Suite 315
Red Bank, NJ 07701
877-986-9472
www.healthywomen.org

Prostate Cancer Foundation (formerly CaPCure)
1250 Fourth Street
Santa Monica, CA 90401
800-757-CURE (757-2873)
310-570-4700
www.prostatecancerfoundation.org

Prostate Forum
P.O. Box 6696
Charlottesville, VA 22906-6696
434-974-1303
www.prostateforum.com

Sexual Dysfunction Association (formerly Impotence Association)
Windmill Place Business Centre
2-4 Windmill Lane
Southall
Middlesex UB2 4NJ
United Kingdom
0870-774-3571
www.sda.uk.net

Sexuality and Developmental Disability Network
Sex Information and Education Council of Canada (SIECCAN)
850 Coxwell Avenue
East York, Ontario, Canada M4C 5RI
416-466-5304
www.sieccan.org

Sexuality Information and Education Council of the United States (SIECUS)
New York Office
130 West 42nd Street, Suite 350
New York, NY 10036
212-819-9770
www.siecus.org

Washington, D.C. Office
1706 R Street NW
Washington, DC 20009
202-265-2405

Us Too! International
5003 Fairview Avenue
Downers Grove, IL 60515
800-80-US TOO (800-808-7866, support hotline)
630-795-1002
www.ustoo.org

Information Available on the Internet Only

Patient Advocates for Advanced Cancer Treatments, Inc. (PAACT)
www.paactusa.org

Phoenix5
www.phoenix5.org

His and Her Health
www.hisandherhealth.com

Prostate Pointers
www.prostatepointers.org

The Sexual Health Network, Inc.
www.sexualhealth.com

Erectile Dysfunction Institute
www.cure-ed.org

Appendix D:
References and Further Reading

Books

Althof, S. E. "Therapeutic Weaving: The Integration of Treatment Techniques," in Stephen B. Levin et al., eds., *Handbook of Clinical Sexuality for Mental Health Professionals.* Brunner-Routledge, 2003.

Anand, Margo. *The Art of Sexual Magic.* G. P. Putnam Sons, New York, 1995.

Angier, Natalie. *Woman, An Intimate Geography.* Houghton Mifflin, New York, 1999.

Bergmann, Martin S. *The Anatomy of Loving.* Fawcett Columbine, New York, 1987.

Block, Joel, D. Ph.D. *Sex over 50.* Parker Publishing Co., West Nyack, N.Y., 1999.

Csikszentmihalyi, Mihaly. *Finding Flow.* BasicBooks, New York, 1997.

Eid, J. François. *Making Love Again: Regaining Sexual Potency.* Brunner-Mazel, New York, 1993.

Eid, J. F. and S. K. Wilson. *Ending E.D.,* privately published, New York.

Ellsworth, Pamela, M.D., J. Heaney, M.D., and C. Gill. *100 Questions & Answers about Prostate Cancer.* Jones and Bartlett Publishers, Sudbury, MA 2003.

Engel, Beverly. *Sensual Sex.* Hunter House, Alameda, Cal., 1999.

Epstein, Gerald, M.D., *Healing Visualizations*. Bantam Books, New York, 1989.

Fisher, Helen. *Anatomy of Love*. Fawcett Columbine, New York, 1992.

Fisher, Helen. *The First Sex*. Ballantine Books, New York, 1999.

Gardner, John W. *Self-Renewal*. Harper Colophon Books, New York, 1963.

Hellstrom, Wayne J. G., M.D., Editor. *The Handbook of Sexual Dysfunction*. The American Society of Andrology, San Francisco, Cal., 1999.

Howe, Desiree Lyon. *His Prostate and Me: A Couple Deals with Prostate Cancer*. Winedale Publishing, London, 2002.

Jacobowitz, Ruth S. *150 Most-Asked Questions about Midlife Sex, Love and Intimacy*. Hearst, New York, 1995.

Jardin, A., G. Wagner, S. Khoury, F. Giuliano, H. Padma-Nathan, R. Rosen *Erectile Dysfunction*. Health Publication Ltd., Plymouth, U.K., 2000.

Joannides, Paul. *The Guide to Getting It On! (The Universe's Coolest and Most Informative Book about Sex)*. Goofy Foot Press, Waldport, Oregon, 2000.

Kirby, R., C. Carson, I. Goldstein. *Erectile Dysfunction*. ISIS Medical Media, Oxford, U.K., 1999.

Kogos, Fred, *1001 Yiddish Proverbs*, Castle Books, Secaucus, N.J., 1974.

Leiblum, Sandra, Ph.D., and Judith Sachs. *Getting the Sex You Want*. ASJA Press, Lincoln, Neb., 2002.

Levinson, Daniel J. *The Seasons of a Man's Life*. Ballantine Books, New York, 1979.

Love, Patricia, Ph.D., and Jo Robinson. *Hot Monogamy*. Plume-Penguin, New York, 1994.

Lue, Tom F., M.D. *Contemporary Diagnosis and Mangement of Male Erectile Dysfunction*. Handbooks in Healthcare Co., Newtown, Penn., 1999.

Masters, William H., and Virginia E. Johnson. *The Pleasure Bond*. Little, Brown, Boston, 1974.

Myers, Charles E., M.D., Sara Steck, R. T., and Rose Myers, P.T., Ph.D., *Eating Your Way to Better Health*. Rivanna Health Publications, Inc., Charlottesville, Va., 2000.

Nicholson, Peggy, *Better Breathing*. PAL Medical, Inc. Maitland, Fla., 1989.

Nerve, the writers at. *The Big Bang: Nerve's Guide to the New Sexual Universe*. Plume, N.Y., 2003.

Ornish, Dean. *Love and Survival*. HarperCollins, New York, 1998.

Otto, H. A. and J. Mann. *Ways of Growth*. Viking Press, New York, 1968.

Padma-Nathan, Harin, M.D. *Medical Management of Erectile Dysfunction: A Primary-Care Manual*. Professional Communications, Inc., 1999.

Penney, Alexandra. *How to Make Love to a Man*. Gramercy Books, New York, 1981.

Pilgrim, Aubrey. *A Revolutionary Approach to Prostate Cancer*. Sterling House, Pittsburgh, Penn., 1998.

Reid, Daniel P. *The Tao of Health, Sex, and Longevity*. Simon & Schuster, New York, 1989.

Ryan, George. *Reclaiming Male Sexuality*. M. Evans, New York, 1997.

Schnarch, David, Ph.D. *Passionate Marriage*. Henry Holt, New York, 1997.

Schnebly, Lee, M.Ed. *Being Happy Being Married*. Fisher Books, Cambridge, Mass., 2001.

Schultz, Susan Polis. *I Keep Falling in Love with You*. Blue Mountain Press, Boulder, Col., 1983.

Schwartz, Richard, M.D. and Jacqueline Olds, M.D. *Marriage in Motion*. Perseus Publishing, Cambridge, Mass., 2000.

Shem, Samuel, M.D., and Janet Surrey, Ph.D. *We Have to Talk*. Basic Books, New York, N.Y., 1998.

Sommer, Frank. *VirgorRobic®, Increased Potency through Specific Fitness Training*. Meyer & Meyer Sport (U.K.) Ltd, Oxford, 2000.

Spark, Richard F., M.D. *Sexual Health for Men*. Perseus Publishing, Cambridge, Mass., 2000.

Strum, Stephen B., M.D., and Donna Pogliano. *A Primer on Prostate Cancer.* Life Extension Media, Hollywood, Fla., 2002.

Vaughan, Susan C., M.D. *Viagra: A Guide to the Phenomenal Potency-Promoting Drug.* Pocket Books, New York, 1998.

Waldman, Mark Robert. *The Art of Staying Together.* Tarcher-Putnam, New York, 1998.

Wallerstein, Judith S. *The Good Marriage: How and Why Love Lasts.* Warner Books, 1996.

Wells, Carol G. *Right Brain Sex.* Prentice Hall Press, New York, 1989.

Scientific and technical papers

Alhof, S. E. When an Erection Alone Is Not Enough: Biopsychological Obstacles to Lovemaking, In *J Impot Res*, 2002 Feb; 14 Suppl. 1:S99–S104.

Brock, Gerald, et al. Safety and Efficacy of Vardenafil for the Treatment of Men with Erectile Dysfunction after Radical Retropubic Prostatectomy, *The Journal of Urology*, 170:1278–1283, October 2003.

Broderick, Gregory A., Craig F. Donatucci, et al. *Male Sexual Dysfunction: Diagnostic and Treatment Options.* American Urological Association, 93rd Annual Meeting, June 1998, 80 pp.

Burnett, Arthur L. Erectile Dysfunction: A Practical Approach for Primary Care, *Geriatrics*, 53(2), February 1998.

Burnett, Arthur L. Neurophysiology of Erectile Function and Dysfunction, *The Handbook of Sexual Dysfunction.* American Society of Andrology, 1999.

Burnett, Arthur L. Strategies to Promote Recovery of Cavernous Nerve Function after Radical Prostatectomy, *World J. Urol.*, 20(2003), 337–342.

Coleman, Craig I., Pharm.D. et al. Vardenafil, *Formulary*, 38:131–148, March 2003.

DeBusk, R., et al., Management of Sexual Dysfunction in Patients with Cardiovascular Disease: Recommendations of the Princeton Consensus Panel (abstract), *American Journal of Cardiology*, 86(2):175–81, July 15, 2000.

DeBusk, R., et al, Management of Sexual Dysfunction in Patients with Cardiovascular Disease: Recommendations of the Princeton Consensus Panel (abstract), *American Journal of Cardiology*, 86(2)Supplement 1:62–68, July 20, 2000.

Donatucci, C. F. Prosexual Drugs: Oral and Topical Agents for Enhancing Erectile and Ejaculatory Control, *Male Sexual Dysfunction: Diagnostic and Treatment Options*. American Urological Association, 1998 Annual Meeting.

Feng, Mark I., S. Huang, et al. Effect of Sildenafil Citrate on Post-Radical Prostatectomy Erectile Dysfunction, *The Journal of Urology*, 164:1935–1938, December 2000.

Geary, E. Stewart, Theresa E. Dendinger, et al. Nerve Sparing Radical Prostatectomy: A Different View, *Journal of Urology*, 154:145–149, July 1995.

Goldstein, Irwin, M.D. et al. Vardenafil, a New Phosphodiesterase Type 5 Inhibitor, in the Treatment of Erectile Dysfunction in Men with Diabetes, *Diabetes Care*, Vol. 26(3): 777–783, March 2003.

Hanash, Kamal A. Comparative Results of Goal Oriented Therapy for Erectile Dysfunction, *Journal of Urology*, 157:2135–2138, June 1997.

Helgason, A. R. et al. Distress Due to Unwanted Side Effects of Prostate Cancer Treatment Is Related to Impaired Well-Being (Quality of Life), *Prostate Cancer and Prostatic Diseases*, 1(3):128, June 1998.

Helgason, Asgeir R. et al. Factors Associated with Waning Sexual Function among Elderly Men and Prostate Cancer Patients, *Journal of Urology*, 158:155–159, July 1997.

Hellstrom, Wayne J. G. et al. Sustained Efficacy and Tolerability of Vardenafil, a Highly Potent Selective Phosphodiesterase Type 5 Inhibitor, in Men with Erectile Dysfunction: Results of a Randomized, Double-Blind, 26-Week Placebo-Controlled Pivotal Trial, *Urology*, 61 (Supplement 4A):8–14, April 2003.

Hellstrom, Wayne J. G. et al. Vardenafil for Treatment of Men with Erectile Dysfunction: Efficacy and Safety in a Randomized, Double-Blind, Placebo-Controlled Trial, *Journal of Andrology*, 23(6):763–771, November–December 2002.

Hopps, C. V. and J. P. Mulhall, Novel Agents for Sexual Dysfunction *BJU International*, 2003.

Incrocci, Luca, M.D., P.C.M. Koper, M.D. et al. Sildenafil Citrate (Viagra) and Erectile Dysfunction Following External Beam Radiotherapy for Prostate Cancer: A Randomized, Double-Blind, Placebo-Controlled, Cross-Over Study, *International Journal of Radiation Oncology: Biology, Physics*, 51(5):1190–1195, 2001.

Jarow, Jonathan P., Patrick Nana-Sinkam et al. Outcome Analysis of Goal Directed Therapy for Impotence, *Journal of Urology*, pp. 1609–12, May 1996.

Kedia, Sumita, C. D. Zippe et al. Treatment of Erectile Dysfunction with Sildenafil Citrate (Viagra) after Radiation Therapy for Prostate Cancer, *Urology*, 54(2):308–312, 1999.

Kim, Edward D., and Larry I. Lipshultz. Advances in the Treatment of Organic Erectile Dysfunction, *Hospital Practice*, April 15, 1997, pp. 101–120.

Kirby, R. S. Medical Management of BPH: Where Are We Going? *Prostate Cancer and Prostatic Diseases*, 2(2):62–65, March 1999.

Kirby, R. S. et al. Prostate Cancer and Sexual Function, *Prostate Cancer and Prostatic Diseases*, 1(4):183, June 1998.

Laumann, Edward O., Anthony Paik et al. Sexual Dysfunction in the United States: Prevalence and Predictors, *Journal of the American Medical Association*, 281(6):537–544.

Litwin, M. S., and D. F. Penson. Health-Related Quality of Life in Men with Prostate Cancer, *Prostate Cancer and Prostatic Diseases*, 1(5):228, June 1998.

Lowentritt, Benjamin H., P. T. Scardino et al. Sildenafil Citrate after Radical Retropubic Prostatectomy, *The Journal of Urology*. 162:1614–1617, November, 1999.

Melman, Arnold. Impotence in the Age of Viagra, *Scientific American Presents*, pp. 62–67, Summer 1999.

Merrick, Gregory S., W. M. Butler et al. Efficacy of Sildenafil Citrate in Prostate Brachytherapy Patients with Erectile Dysfunction, *Urology*, 53(6):1112–1116, 1999.

Morales, Alvaro, Jeremy P. W. Heaton et al. Oral and Topical Treatment of Erectile Dysfunction: Present and Future, *Urologic Clinics of North America,* 22(4):879–886, November 1995.

Mulhall, John P. Deciphering Erectile Dysfunction Drug Trials, *The Journal of Urology,* 170:353-358, August 2003

Myers, Robert P. Editorial: Prostate Cancer—Neurovascular Preservation; Smoking Cessation May Enhance Prognosis? *The Journal of Urology,* 154:158–159, July 1995.

National Institutes of Health, Impotence, *NIH Consensus Statement Online,* National Institutes of Health, 10(4):1–31, December 7–9, 1992.

Nehra, Ajay. Oxygen Levels and Their Effect on Erectile Function, *Family Urology,* p. 19, Winter 1997.

Padma-Nathan, H, V. J. Stecher et al. Minimal Time to Successful Intercourse after Sildenafil Citrate: Results of a Randomized, Double-Blind, Placebo-Controlled Trial, *Urology,* 62(3):400–403, 2003.

Padma-Nathan, H, C. Steidle et al. The Efficacy and Safety of a Topical Alprostadil Cream, Alprox-TD®, for the Treatment of Erectile Dysfunction: Two Phase 2 Studies in Mild-to-Moderate and Severe ED, *International Journal of Importance Research,* 15(1):10–17, February 2003.

Penson, D. F. Transitions in Health-Related Quality of Life during the First Nine Months after Diagnosis with Prostate Cancer, *Prostate Cancer and Prostatic Diseases,* 1(3):134, June 1998.

Porst, H. Padma-Nathan, H. et. al. Efficacy of Tadalafil for the Treatment of Erectile Dysfunction at 24 and 36 Hours after Dosing: a Randomized Controlled Trial (abstract), *Urology,* 62(1):121–125, 2003.

Quinlan, David M., Jonathan I. Epstein et al. Sexual Function Following Radical Prostatectomy: Influence of Preservation of Neurovascular Bundles, *Journal of Urology,* 145, 998–1002.

Raina, Rupesh, M. M. Lakin et al. Long-Term Effect of Sildenafil Citrate on Erectile Dysfunction after Radical Prostatectomy: 3-Year Follow-Up, *Urology,* 62(1):110–115, 2003.

Rosen, Raymond, Ph.D., Irwin Goldstein et al. *A Process of Care Model*, The University of Medicine and Dentistry (UMDNJ)-Robert Wood Johnson Medical School, 1998.

Sadovsky, R. Managing Sexual Dysfunction in Cardiac Patients, *American Family Physician*, December 1, 2000.

Schover, Leslie R., Ph.D. Sexual Rehabilitation after Treatment for Prostate Cancer, *Cancer Supplement*, 71(3):1024–1030, February 1, 1993.

Shabsigh, R., H. Padma-Nathan et al. Intracavernous Alprostadil Alfadex Is More Efficacious, Better Tolerated, and Preferred over Intraurethral Alprostadil Plus Optional Actis: A Comparative, Randomized, Crossover, Multicenter Study, *Urology*, 55(1):109–113, 2000.

Shabsigh, R., H. Padma-Nathta et al. Intracavernous Alprostadil Alfaces (EDEX/VIRIDAL) is Effective and Safe in Patients with Erectile Dysfunction after Failing Sildenafil (Viagra), *Urology*, 55(4):477–480, 2000.

Sommer, F. et al. Creative-dynamic Image Synthesis: A Useful Addition to the Treatment Options for Impotence, *International Journal of Impotence Research*, 13:268–275 2001.

Thadani, Udho, M.D. et al. The Effect of Vardenafil, a Potent and Highly Selective Phosphodiesterase-5 Inhibitor for the Treatment of Erectile Dysfunction, on the Cardiovascular Response to Exercise in Patients with Coronary Artery Disease, *Journal of the American College of Cardiology*, 40(11):2006–2012, December 4, 2002.

Zagaja, Gregory P., D. A. Mhoon et al. Sildenafil in the Treatment of Erectile Dysfunction after Radical Prostatectomy, *Urology*, 56(4):631–934, 2000.

Zelefsky, Michael J., A. B. Mckee, H. Lee, and S. A. Leibel. Efficacy of Oral Sildenafil in Patients with Erectile Dysfunction after Radiotherapy for Carcinoma of the Prostate, *Urology*, 53(4):775–777, 1999.

Zippe, Craig D. F. M. Jhaveri et al. Role of Viagra after Radical Prostatectomy, *Urology*, 55(2):241–245, 2000.

Zonszein, Joel. Diagnosis and Management of Endocrine Disorders of Erectile Dysfunction, *Urologic Clinics of North America*, 22(4):789–802, November 1995.

Index

See also "Appendix D: References and Further Reading" (pages 205–212).

depression, as cause for lack of desire, 43
desire, increasing, 43–45
Desyrel, 193
devices, 147–156
diabetes:
  as cause of erectile dysfunction, 12
  prevention of, 80–81
Diamond, Neil, 38
dietary supplements, in treatment of erectile dysfunction, 178–180
differences, handling, 34–35
disease, as cause of erectile dysfunction, 12
doctor:
  talking with, 89–96
  understanding situation of, 90–91
"domestic" sex, 38
dopamine receptor agonists, 178
Dostinex, 178, 193
doxazosin, used in combination with Viagra®, 175
drugs:
  as cause of erectile dysfunction, 12–13
  purchase of, from non-U.S. sources, 105
"Dunlop's disease," 81

earlobe, as touchpoint, 69
eating right, 81–82
Eating Your Way to Better Health (Myers), 82
ED, *see* erectile dysfunction
ED cocktails, *see* erection cocktails
EDEX®, 128, 138, 190
  information, 140–141
  www.edex.com, 141
Education Center for Prostate Cancer Patients (ECPCP, *www.ecpcp.org*), 202
Elephant Syndrome, 25–28
Encore Medical Products (*www.impoaid.com*), xvi, 150, 153, 191
  products and contact information, 196
Endocare, *see* Timm Medical Technology
Engle, Beverly, 72, 73
ErecAid™ Esteem™ System, 150, 156, 191
  information, 156
  www.timmmedical.com, 156
erection (*see also* impotence):
  having loving and satisfying sexual relationship without, 6–9
  importance of, to partner, 52–53
  need for, in orgasm, 21
  nerves for, 47–48
  as result of penile injection, 135
"erection cocktails," for treatment of erectile dysfunction, 100, 174–177

erectile dysfunction:
  causes of 12–13
  in context of couple's relationship, 24–25
  discussing with doctor, 91–93
  discussing with new partner, 34
  mindset, breaking, 6–7, 10
  possibility of, after cancer therapy, 4, 17–18
  relationship with exercise, 84
  research, 169–171
  and sensual dysfunction, 61
  synonymous with "impotence," 12
  therapies for, 97–171
Erectile Dysfunction Institute (*www.cure-ed.org*), 204
exercise information online (*www.cdc.gov, www.fpnotebook.com, www.walking.about.com, www.men-and-health.info*), 85–87
exercising, 82–88

face, as touchpoint, 68
feet, as touchpoints, 69
Food and Drug Administration (FDA), 104, 126, 174
Friedman School of Nutrition Science and Policy at Tufts University, 84

Garrity, Joan Terry, 72
generic drugs, purchase of, from non-U.S. sources, 105–106
genital area, as touchpoint, 70
getting into shape, 79–88
gingko, 180–181
GlaxoSmithKline, 116
goals, setting, as step in improving relationship, 30
Goldstein, Dr. Irwin, 84, 168
Good Marriage, The: How and Why Love Lasts (Wallerstein), 5
GPI 1485, 144, 194
  information, 145
  www.guilfordpharm.com, 145
gravity, use of, to overcome impotency, 75
Guilford Pharmaceuticals, 144, 145, 167

habituation, defined, 5
hands, as touchpoints, 69
head of penis, as touchpoint, 70
heart disease, prevention of, 80
heart-to-heart talk, as step in improving relationship, 31–32

CPSIA information can be obtained
at www.ICGtesting.com
Printed in the USA
FFOW02n1321130618
47128734-49670FF

9 780738 207896